VACCINES AND YOUR FAMILY

VACCINES & YOUR FAMILY

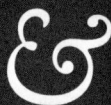

COLUMBIA
UNIVERSITY
PRESS

NEW YORK

*Separating Fact
from Fiction*

PAUL A. OFFIT, MD, FAAP
and CHARLOTTE A. MOSER, MS

The information in this book is not intended to replace the medical care or advice you receive from your doctor. You are encouraged to consult your family physician or pediatrician on all matters concerning your family's health and to follow their advice. This book was completed in February 2024, and the information is correct as of this date. As new findings become available through research, some of the recommendations herein might be subject to change. You are encouraged to seek the most up-to-date information on vaccinations from your family's health care providers. In addition, you will find numerous websites in this book that can provide accurate and up-to-date information on all aspects of vaccination.

COLUMBIA UNIVERSITY PRESS
Publishers Since 1893
New York   Chichester, West Sussex

cup.columbia.edu
Copyright © 2024 Paul A. Offit and Charlotte A. Moser

First edition published as *Vaccines and Your Child: Separating Fact from Fiction*, 2011
All rights reserved

Library of Congress Cataloging-in-Publication Data
Names: Offit, Paul A., author. | Moser, Charlotte A., author.
Title: Vaccines and your family : separating fact from fiction /
    Paul A. Offit and Charlotte A. Moser.
Description: New York : Columbia University Press, [2024] |
    Includes bibliographical references and index.
Identifiers: LCCN 2023057327 (print) | LCCN 2023057328 (ebook) |
    ISBN 9780231213387 (hardback) | ISBN 9780231213394 (trade paperback) |
    ISBN 9780231559867 (ebook)
Subjects: LCSH: Vaccination—Popular works. | Vaccines—Popular works. |
    Vaccination of children—Popular works.
Classification: LCC RA638 .O335 2024 (print) | LCC RA638 (ebook) |
    DDC 614.4/7—dc23/eng/20240301
LC record available at https://lccn.loc.gov/2023057327
LC ebook record available at https://lccn.loc.gov/2023057328

Printed in the United States of America

Cover design: Noah Arlow
Cover image: iStock

CONTENTS

VACCINES AND YOUR FAMILY

QUESTIONS PEOPLE HAVE ABOUT VACCINES

GENERAL QUESTIONS

WHAT ARE VACCINES?

Vaccines provide the immunity that comes from natural infection without the consequences of natural infection.

One way to understand vaccines is to examine the origins of the first one: the smallpox vaccine. In the late 1700s, Edward Jenner, a physician working in southern England, noticed that milkmaids didn't catch smallpox, a disease that swept across the English countryside every two to three years. Jenner believed there was a connection between the blisters milkmaids often suffered on their hands—blisters like those on cows' udders—and protection against disease. He reasoned that the blisters must contain something protective. He tested his theory by taking fluid from a blister (pus) on the wrist of a milkmaid named Sarah Nelmes and injecting it into the arm of a local laborer's son named James Phipps. Then Jenner did something that would never pass an ethical review board today. A few weeks later, he injected the boy with dried pus taken from someone who had smallpox. Phipps survived. Jenner had shown that pus from the milkmaid's blister (now known to contain cowpox) had protected Phipps from human smallpox.

Jenner's vaccine worked because he had unknowingly taken advantage of what we now call species barriers. Viruses or bacteria that have adapted over centuries to infecting one species often aren't very good at infecting another. This worked to Jenner's advantage. Although cowpox doesn't cause disease in people, it still causes an immune response. And fortunately, the two viruses—cowpox and smallpox—are similar enough that immunization with one protects against disease from the other. In this book, we'll talk about the many ways vaccines provide protection against disease without causing disease.

Jenner was way ahead of his time. Today, we know that cowpox and smallpox are viruses, but Jenner didn't know that. In fact, he didn't know what germs were; the germ theory (i.e., that specific germs can cause specific diseases) wouldn't be postulated for a hundred years. So, Jenner's observations were pure phenomenology. But he was right. And smallpox, a disease that killed as many as five hundred million people—more than any other infectious disease—has been eliminated from the face of the earth. A remarkable achievement.

DID YOU KNOW?

Jenner also contributed something else: the word *vaccine*. Because his smallpox vaccine was derived from a cow, he described it using the Latin word *vaccinae*, meaning "of the cow." Today, although only a couple vaccines are derived from bacteria or viruses that infect cows, they are all still called vaccines.

Reference

Tucker, Jonathan B. *Scourge: The Once and Future Threat of Smallpox.* New York: Atlantic Monthly, 2001.

WHY DO WE STILL NEED VACCINES?

The only vaccine discontinued because the disease it protected against was eliminated from the face of the earth is the smallpox vaccine. That's it—just one. All other vaccine-preventable diseases still cause suffering and death in the United States, elsewhere in the world, or both. Vaccines continue to be necessary for several reasons.

Some diseases still occur commonly in the United States. Several vaccine-preventable diseases are still common: chickenpox (varicella), pertussis (whooping cough), pneumococcus, hepatitis A, hepatitis B, rotavirus, influenza, meningococcus, and human papillomavirus (HPV). All these diseases can make us seriously ill or even kill us.

The chickenpox vaccine was introduced in 1995. At the time, about four million cases of chickenpox occurred in the United States every year. Within a few years, that number declined to about four hundred thousand—a 90 percent drop. However, although one dose of the vaccine protected 95 of 100 people from getting very sick, it only protected 80 of 100 from getting a mild form of the disease. And people with mild disease are still contagious. To increase protection against mild disease from 80 to 95 percent, a second dose of vaccine was recommended. The use of a second dose has decreased the incidence of disease even more, but we still have a way to go to eliminate chickenpox.

A vaccine to prevent pneumococcus, a disease that occurs commonly in young children, was introduced in 2000. Consequently, childhood infections caused by pneumococcus, which include meningitis, pneumonia (lung inflammation), and bloodstream infections, have been dramatically reduced. But they haven't been eliminated; thousands of children still experience pneumococcal infections every year. Likewise, pneumococcus continues to infect thousands of older and high-risk adults each year. So, it's still important to get the vaccine.

Because a pertussis vaccine has been around since the 1940s, it might surprise you to know that the disease is still quite common. Every year hundreds of thousands of adolescents, teens, and adults catch and transmit pertussis. That's because immunity to pertussis wanes. Before the vaccine, every year about seven thousand people died from pertussis; most were young infants. Today, fewer than thirty infants die each year from the disease, so the vaccine has been quite effective. But because immunity fades, adolescents and young adults are at risk; fortunately, a vaccine to protect adolescents and adults became available in 2005. But we still have a long way to go before we eliminate pertussis.

Hepatitis A virus—which causes severe, but rarely fatal, liver infection—can be transmitted by contaminated food. An outbreak of hepatitis A at a Mexican restaurant in western Pennsylvania in 2003 sickened more than six hundred people, and four died. Several more recent outbreaks have been traced to fresh or frozen foods purchased at grocery stores. The virus still infects thousands of people every year.

Hepatitis B virus infections are particularly difficult to eliminate because they're so long-lived. About a million people in the United States are chronically infected with the virus. Many people with chronic infections don't have any symptoms and therefore don't know they're sick, but they're still contagious.

A vaccine to prevent rotavirus, which causes fever, vomiting, and diarrhea in young children, has been used in the United States since 2006. During the next few years, the annual number of rotavirus infections dropped from about three million to fewer than three hundred thousand. It is now very rare for children to be hospitalized for dehydration caused by this virus, but rotavirus continues to circulate. For these reasons, the rotavirus vaccine is still worth getting.

Influenza is unusual in that it requires a vaccine to be given every year. Because tens of thousands of people are hospitalized with influenza pneumonia each year, and because the virus changes enough that immunization or natural infection in one year doesn't protect against disease the following year, the choice to get an influenza vaccine should be an easy one.

The HPV vaccine was recommended for all young women in 2006 and for young men in 2009. The vaccine prevents several cancers, including the only known cause of cervical cancer, a disease that occurs about twenty to twenty-five years after initially being infected. About 70 percent of women will catch HPV within five years of their first sexual encounter. It's very difficult to avoid this virus.

Some diseases still occur in the United States but are uncommon. Some vaccine-preventable diseases, like measles, mumps, tetanus, *Haemophilus influenzae* type b (Hib), and meningococcus still occur in the United States but less frequently than those just mentioned. Measles and Hib typically cause disease in fewer than a hundred children every year, mumps and meningococcus in several hundred.

Although these diseases are uncommon, they can be devastating. One measles outbreak in California is a perfect example. In 2008, a San Diego family took their unvaccinated children on vacation to Switzerland, where one caught measles. (Measles occurs fairly commonly in Western Europe, where immunization rates aren't very high.) The child brought the disease home with him and proceeded to infect several children waiting in the pediatrician's office, one of whom developed severe dehydration. The disease also spread to classmates and people with whom he had come into contact at a grocery store. All those infected were unvaccinated. A similar measles epidemic occurred in Southern California in 2015. Most people don't realize that every year about sixty people with measles enter the United States, primarily from Western Europe. Typically, because most Americans are immunized, the virus doesn't spread. But the outbreaks in California show that when enough people choose not to vaccinate their children, the virus can spread rapidly. So, the choice not to have one's children vaccinated against measles is a very real choice to risk their getting this disease that, before the introduction of a vaccine in 1963, annually caused about forty-eight thousand children to be hospitalized with pneumonia or encephalitis (a brain infection) and about five hundred to die.

Some diseases have been virtually eliminated from the United States but still occur in other parts of the world. One vaccine-preventable disease, polio, was eliminated in the Western Hemisphere by the late 1970s. Another disease, diphtheria, causes fewer than five infections in the United States every year. Although polio and diphtheria have been completely or virtually eliminated, respectively, from the United States, they haven't been eliminated from the world. Polio still infects people in several countries, and diphtheria infections occur in many countries. Because international travel is common, it's likely that if enough people choose not to vaccinate, these diseases will be back. And that's exactly what happened during the dissolution of the Soviet Union in the early 1990s when, because of a severe drop in immunization rates, tens of thousands of children suffered diphtheria, and thousands died.

Reference
Orenstein, Walter A., Paul A. Offit, Kathryn M. Edwards, and Stanley A. Plotkin, eds. *Plotkin's Vaccines*, 8th ed. London: Elsevier, 2024.

HOW DO VACCINES WORK?

Let's use the measles vaccine as an example. Before the measles vaccine became available in 1963, millions of American children got measles every year. The virus is transmitted from one person to another by sneezing, coughing, or talking. Once it enters the nose and throat, the virus reproduces over and over again. In a few days, hundreds of viruses become millions of viruses, causing rash, fever, cough, red eyes, and a runny nose.

During infection, the immune system recognizes measles viruses as foreign and attacks them. The most important part of the attack is the formation of antibodies, which are proteins in the bloodstream that bind to viruses and neutralize them, causing the disease to subside. Better still, measles antibodies protect the person from this disease for the rest of their life. A natural measles infection induces lifelong protective immunity. Antibodies are the key to this protection.

DID YOU KNOW?

The immune response involves many types of cells that fight infection. But in the world of vaccines, one important component of the immune response is antibodies, which neutralize viruses and bacteria before infections can develop.

Although the goal of a vaccine is to induce the same quantity of protective antibodies as would be induced by natural infection, this rarely happens. Nothing is better than natural infection for inducing an effective immune response. But the problem with natural infection is that children must often pay a high price for immunity. The goal of a measles vaccine is to prevent all this suffering, hospitalization, and death. But when the measles vaccine was first used, it was unclear whether it could induce an immune response similar enough to that of natural infection to provide lifelong protection. Several decades would pass before this question was answered. But then the answer was clear.

Whereas the natural measles virus reproduces thousands of times, the measles vaccine virus reproduces fewer than a hundred times. This means that the quantity of antibodies induced by vaccination is less than that induced by natural infection, about a third less. Fortunately, that's good enough. Because of the measles vaccine, the number of children infected with measles virus every year has declined from millions to fewer than a hundred, almost all of whom are unvaccinated. The number of children hospitalized for measles in the United States is now very small. The measles vaccine did what it was supposed to do: it induced an immune response similar enough to that of natural infection to protect children without subjecting them to the occasionally deadly consequences of natural infection.

The story of the measles vaccine has been repeated for every other vaccine. Although the immune response to vaccines is typically less than that of natural infection, it's more than adequate to prevent much of the suffering and death caused by the diseases each protects against.

HOW ARE VACCINES MADE?

All vaccines are made with the same goal in mind: to separate the virulent parts of the virus or bacterium (i.e., the parts that make you sick) from the immunogenic parts (i.e., the parts that induce a protective immune response). Different processes are used depending on whether the disease is caused by viruses or bacteria.

Viral Vaccines

A viral vaccine is made using one of four strategies.

Weaken the virus. One way to make a viral vaccine is to weaken the virus, so that it cannot reproduce enough to cause disease, but it still reproduces enough to induce a protective immune response. It's a fine line. And it's not very easy to do. But it has been accomplished for several viruses: measles, mumps, rubella, chickenpox, influenza, and rotavirus.

The strategy for making the measles, mumps, and chickenpox vaccines, as well as one of the rotavirus vaccines (Rotarix), is the same. It was pioneered by Max Theiler, a researcher working at the Rockefeller Institute in New York City in the 1930s. Theiler knew that viruses only reproduce in cells (unlike bacteria, which do not need cells to reproduce). He also knew that human viruses grow better in human cells than in nonhuman cells. Thus, Theiler reasoned that if he could adapt human viruses to grow in nonhuman cells (like those of chickens or mice), he could weaken the viruses' ability to grow in human cells. Theiler made the first live, weakened human vaccine in 1935, one that protected against a disease that killed hundreds of thousands of people in South America as well as many Americans working on the Panama Canal: yellow fever. Theiler weakened yellow fever virus by growing it many times in chicken and mouse cells. For his efforts, he was awarded the Nobel Prize in Physiology or Medicine in 1951. Following Theiler's lead, researchers found that the measles and mumps viruses are weakened by growth in chicken embryo cells, the chickenpox virus by growth in guinea pig cells, and rotavirus by growth in monkey kidney cells.

Another way to weaken viruses is to grow them at temperatures lower than body temperature. This strategy has been used to make the rubella and nasal-spray influenza (FluMist) vaccines. In both cases, these viruses no longer reproduce themselves well at body temperature, so they cannot cause disease. But they reproduce well enough to induce a protective immune response.

A further way to weaken a virus is a modification of the method used by Edward Jenner when he made the smallpox vaccine: take advantage of species barriers (see "What Are Vaccines?"). That is how one of the rotavirus vaccines (RotaTeq) is made. RotaTeq contains parts of a cow rotavirus that doesn't reproduce well in people along with parts of human rotaviruses that are necessary to induce a protective immune response. This vaccine represents the best of two worlds: it retains the weakened virulence characteristics of the cow rotavirus, yet it also contains the human components necessary to induce protective immunity.

Inactivate the virus. Another way to make a viral vaccine is to kill the virus with a chemical, typically a small amount of formaldehyde (see "Do Vaccines Contain Harmful Chemicals Like Formaldehyde?"). Unlike weakened viral vaccines—in which viruses continue to reproduce a little—killed viruses can't reproduce at all. However, the human body still reacts to an inactivated virus and mounts a protective immune response. This is how the hepatitis A and polio vaccines are made.

Use only part of the virus. A viral vaccine can also be made by using just one viral protein.

Viruses are made of proteins. Some viruses are small, like hepatitis A virus, and contain only a few proteins. And some viruses are large, like chickenpox, which contains about seventy proteins. (The largest mammalian virus is smallpox, which has about two hundred proteins.) The strategy of using only one viral protein to make a vaccine works only if that protein is principally responsible for inducing a protective immune response. Four viral vaccines work this way: those for hepatitis B, HPV, and respiratory syncytial virus (RSV), as well as one for COVID-19 (Novavax). Each is made using recombinant DNA technology.

Recombinant DNA technology was first used to make medical products in the 1970s, the first of which was insulin. By the late 1980s, this technology was being used to make a vaccine: hepatitis B. Researchers used the gene that made one hepatitis B protein, called hepatitis B surface protein, because they knew that an immune response against it could protect people against disease. Then, they put the gene that made this protein into a plasmid, a small circular piece of DNA. The plasmid they chose reproduced itself in yeast. Next, they put the yeast plasmid containing the hepatitis B gene into common baker's yeast. As the yeast cells reproduced, the plasmid also reproduced and made the hepatitis B surface protein, which was later purified to make the vaccine. The HPV vaccine is also made in yeast cells. The protein in the COVID-19 vaccine (made by Novavax) is produced in insect cells.

Administer the gene that codes for one viral protein. The messenger RNA (mRNA) COVID-19 vaccines made by Pfizer and Moderna also rely on just a single protein—the spike protein—from SARS-CoV-2, the virus that causes COVID-19. However, instead of delivering the viral protein directly, these vaccines deliver the gene that codes for the protein. The gene, known as mRNA, enters cells and uses the cells' own machinery to manufacture the SARS-CoV-2 spike protein. While all other viral vaccine strategies use some form of the virus, mRNA vaccines rely on the body of the inoculated person to do two things: first, make the viral protein; second, induce an immune response against that protein.

Bacterial Vaccines

Because bacteria are far more complex than viruses, the processes used to make bacterial vaccines are different from those used to make viral vaccines. Three strategies are used.

Use the sugar that coats the bacterial surface. Bacteria are much bigger than viruses. Whereas the largest virus, smallpox, contains about two hundred proteins, the smallest bacteria contain more than two thousand proteins—and most contain between three thousand and four thousand proteins. Fortunately, the protective immune responses to several bacteria that cause disease aren't directed against bacterial proteins. Rather, they're directed against a polysaccharide, a complex sugar that coats the surface of the bacteria. Researchers were able to make some bacterial vaccines using the bacterial polysaccharide only. But in most cases, the polysaccharide is conjugated (linked) to a harmless protein to enhance the immune response. This is how the pneumococcal, meningococcal, and *Haemophilus influenzae* type b (Hib) vaccines are made.

Inactivate the bacterial toxin. Some bacteria cause disease by making harmful toxins. For vaccines against this type of bacteria, researchers inactivate the toxins with a chemical (like formaldehyde), rendering the toxins harmless but still capable of inducing protection. (Inactivated toxins are called toxoids.) Diphtheria and tetanus vaccines are made using this strategy; each makes a single toxin that causes disease.

Purify bacterial proteins. One bacterial vaccine stands alone for its use of two strategies: the pertussis (or whooping cough) vaccine. To make pertussis vaccine, researchers purify several critical proteins needed to induce a protective immune response. These purified proteins are then treated with formaldehyde to render them harmless. Some of these proteins are toxins (as in the diphtheria and tetanus vaccines), and some are part of the bacterial structure. Several pertussis vaccines are available, each containing between two and five pertussis proteins.

References

Offit, Paul A. *Vaccinated: One Man's Quest to Defeat the World's Deadliest Diseases.* New York: Smithsonian, 2007.
Orenstein, Walter A., Paul A. Offit, Kathryn M. Edwards, and Stanley A. Plotkin, eds. *Plotkin's Vaccines,* 8th ed. London: Elsevier, 2024.

HOW DO PHARMACEUTICAL COMPANIES MAKE VACCINES?

Vaccine manufacturing is a long process with many steps. Most people don't realize that it can take years and cost hundreds of millions of dollars. One rotavirus vaccine licensed by the Food and Drug Administration (FDA) in 2006 is a good example of what it takes to develop a modern vaccine.

Between 1979 and 1990, researchers at the Children's Hospital of Philadelphia and the Wistar Institute created the five strains of rotavirus that eventually became the RotaTeq vaccine. The strains were then licensed to a pharmaceutical company so they could do the large-scale and expensive studies needed to develop the vaccine. For example, the pharmaceutical company did studies to determine exactly how much vaccine virus should be in the final product. Too much might cause unwanted side effects; too little would be insufficient to induce protection.

The pharmaceutical company then had to establish how many doses of vaccine were needed to induce an effective immune response. This meant studying thousands of children given different numbers of doses. The company then had to prove that all vials contained the same amount of vaccine.

The company also had to prove that the vaccine didn't contain contaminating agents that could infect people, like other viruses or bacteria, parasites, or fungi. This meant hundreds and hundreds more tests, called adventitious-agent testing. (In 2010, a powerful new technology called deep sequencing was developed to detect minute quantities of bacterial or viral genes in vaccines).

The company then had to buffer the vaccine to prolong its shelf life and stabilize it so that the vaccine viruses were distributed equally throughout each vial and wouldn't interfere with one another. And scientists at the company had to figure out whether the vaccine should be placed in plastic or glass vials, depending on which material would provide the longest shelf life and would better prevent the vaccine viruses from sticking to the sides of the vial.

Next came the hardest and most expensive part: proving that the vaccine worked and was safe. This meant studying more than seventy thousand children in twelve countries for four years. Half the children got the vaccine by mouth at two, four, and six months of age, and the other half were given a placebo, a fluid provided in the same type of vial as the vaccine with the same buffering and stabilizing agents but without any vaccine viruses. This trial, which cost about $350 million, created an amount of paperwork that, if stacked one sheet on top of another, would exceed the height of the Willis Tower (formerly the Sears Tower) in Chicago.

Finally, the pharmaceutical company had to conduct what are called concomitant-use studies to prove that their new vaccine didn't interfere with the safety or immune responses of other vaccines that would be given at the same time and that existing vaccines didn't interfere with the safety or immune responses of their new vaccine. These studies were enormously laborious and expensive. When they were completed, after sixteen years and at a cost of about $1 billion, the company submitted their findings and request for approval to the FDA. The filing contained enough paperwork to fill the back of a small U-Haul truck.

Reference

Vesikari, Timo, David O. Matson, Penelope Dennehy, et al. "Safety and Efficacy of a Pentavalent Human-Bovine (WC3) Reassortant Rotavirus Vaccine." *New England Journal of Medicine* 354, no. 1 (2006): 23–33.

HOW ARE VACCINES RECOMMENDED?

A vaccine recommendation involves three steps.

Licensure

First, vaccines must be licensed. Before investigators at a pharmaceutical company test a vaccine, they must obtain an Investigational New Drug (IND) license from the FDA. An IND license is awarded only if the company has shown that the vaccine, when tested in experimental animals, is safe and induces an immune response likely to be protective. The company must also show that the vaccine is made according to Good Manufacturing Practices (GMP), which ensure it is free from contaminating microorganisms that could be harmful.

Once an IND license is obtained, the pharmaceutical company tests the vaccine in progressively larger numbers of adults, teenagers, and children to make sure that it works. Even if young children are the intended recipients of the vaccine, these studies, which can take as long as twenty years, almost always begin in small numbers of healthy adults before progressing to teens and then to older and younger children. The results of the studies are then submitted to the FDA in the form of a biologics license application (BLA) for a vaccine license. The FDA's decision is based on two factors: safety and efficacy. The licensure process takes about ten months. Once a vaccine is licensed, pharmaceutical companies have the right to sell it.

Recommendation

Second, the vaccine must be recommended. Even after the FDA has licensed a vaccine, doctors wait until the vaccine is recommended before giving it to their patients.

Several committees recommend vaccines, including the Advisory Committee on Immunization Practices, which advises the Centers for Disease Control and Prevention (CDC); the

Committee on Infectious Diseases, which advises the American Academy of Pediatrics (AAP); and the American Academy of Family Physicians, among others. Each advisory body is composed of ten to fifteen physicians and scientists with extensive experience in infectious diseases, epidemiology, immunology, and microbiology. The issues considered by these groups are somewhat different from those considered by the FDA. Whereas the FDA considers whether a vaccine is safe and effective, recommendations are based on whether a vaccine would be useful as part of the broader public health policy.

Requirement

Third, some vaccines are required for admission to day care, elementary school, middle school, high school, and even college. These requirements, or mandates, are state based and often determined by what states and localities can afford. The federal government doesn't mandate vaccines.

From a parent's perspective, the only information that should matter is whether a vaccine is safe and effective and whether it has been recommended. In other words, vaccine recommendations are more important to making informed health decisions than vaccine requirements.

DID YOU KNOW?

Unfortunately, many parents and even some doctors focus only on which vaccines are required, not which ones are recommended. In some cases, families affected by vaccine-preventable diseases, such as bacterial meningitis, have said they didn't know that a vaccine was recommended and assumed that because it wasn't required it wasn't necessary.

HOW DO WE KNOW VACCINES WORK?

We live longer than we used to.

During the twentieth century, the average American life span increased by thirty years. Antibiotics, purified drinking water, sanitation, safer workplaces, better nutrition, safer foods, seatbelts, and a decline in smoking accounted for some of that increase. But no single medical advance has had a greater impact on improving human health than vaccines.

Before vaccines, Americans could expect the following every year:

- Measles would infect four million children and kill five hundred.
- Diphtheria would kill thousands of people, mostly young children.
- Rubella would cause as many as twenty thousand babies to be born blind or deaf or to suffer mental delays.
- Pertussis would kill seven thousand children, most less than one year old.
- Polio would permanently paralyze fifteen thousand children and kill one thousand.

Because of vaccines, some of these diseases have been completely or virtually eliminated from the United States. Smallpox—a disease estimated to have killed 500 million people—was completely eradicated by vaccines.

Although most pediatricians today didn't witness firsthand the decline of diseases like diphtheria, smallpox, or pertussis, they did witness the virtual elimination of one bacterial infection: *Haemophilus influenzae* type b (Hib). Before the vaccine, Hib caused about twenty-five thousand children a year to suffer meningitis, bloodstream infections, and pneumonia. Because of the Hib vaccine, first used in the early 1990s, fewer than one hundred children are now affected annually.

Reference

Bunker, John P., Howard S. Frazier, and Frederick Mosteller. "Improving Health: Measuring Effects of Medical Care." *Milbank Quarterly* 72, no. 2 (1994): 225–58.

ARE VACCINE-PREVENTABLE DISEASES REALLY THAT BAD?

Parents who choose not to vaccinate their children or choose to delay or withhold vaccines are taking a risk. It's not a big risk; in fact, the odds are in their favor. In all likelihood, their children will not suffer permanent harm or die from an infectious disease. Polio has been eliminated from the United States; so has rubella. Diphtheria occurs in only a few people a year. And although measles cases occur every year in the United States, and we witnessed significant measles epidemics in 2015 and 2019, no one died. So what's the harm of not vaccinating?

The fact is that every year vaccine-preventable diseases still kill children in the United States. Influenza typically kills about one hundred children a year. HPV is a long-range killer, causing fatal cervical, anal, and oral cancers years after initial infection. Pneumococcus and meningococcus, both of which cause meningitis, leave many children permanently disabled. If the trend of not vaccinating or delaying vaccination continues, other diseases—like polio and diphtheria—will be back. Indeed, in June 2022, in Rockland County, New York, a twenty-seven-year-old man who had not left the United States was paralyzed by poliovirus.

Probably those best suited to explaining why vaccines are important are those who belong to advocacy organizations, like Families Fighting Flu, Meningitis Angels, American Society for Meningitis Prevention, and Cervivor, all of whom tell similar stories. They or their children were healthy and active until they were killed or had the course of their life altered by a vaccine-preventable disease. Often, they say that they thought it couldn't happen to them—until it did. Some of them become crusaders to prevent others from having to live their horror.

Choosing not to vaccinate is like playing Russian roulette, except instead of having a gun with five empty chambers and one bullet, it's a gun with hundreds of thousands of empty chambers and one bullet. But why take the chance? Why play the game at all if you don't have to? People who belong to these advocacy groups ask themselves that question every day. The problem is that they never realized they *were* taking a risk. In some cases, they didn't know there was a vaccine; in others, they just thought it wasn't necessary. One reason that doctors are passionate about vaccines is that they see people with diseases like pertussis, chickenpox, pneumococcus, and meningococcus. They know what it looks like to be sick, to suffer, and to die from these infections. That's why it's so hard for them to send unvaccinated or undervaccinated patients out of their offices: they know what being unprotected could mean.

References

Cervivor: https://cervivor.org
Families Fighting Flu: http://www.familiesfightingflu.org
Meningitis Angels: http://www.meningitis-angels.org
American Society for Meningitis Prevention: https://meningitisprevention.org/

ARE VACCINES GIVEN AS ONE SIZE FITS ALL?

Some people wonder how the same vaccine can be recommended for a ten-pound baby and a two-hundred-pound adult. Wouldn't it make more sense to give a baby a smaller amount of vaccine? That's what is done for drugs, where the amount prescribed is often determined by weight or age.

Indeed, some vaccine doses given to children and adults aren't the same. For example, the hepatitis B vaccine given to children contains less vaccine than the one given to adults. But sometimes the opposite is true. For example, the amount of diphtheria and pertussis vaccine in the DTaP vaccine given to children is more than is in the Tdap vaccine given to adolescents and adults (see the section on "Diphtheria, Tetanus, and Pertussis"). That's because adolescents and adults often have more serious local reactions to the diphtheria and pertussis components of the vaccine than children do.

But the importance of weight in relation to dose isn't the same for vaccines as it is for drugs. Drugs enter the bloodstream and are distributed throughout the body. That's not true for vaccines. With a few exceptions, such as the intranasal influenza vaccine and the orally administered rotavirus vaccine, most vaccines are typically injected into the arm, leg, or buttocks. Regardless of how a vaccine is administered, the part that generates immunity, called the antigen, is transported to nearby lymph nodes, which are collections of immune cells located throughout the body. Transport occurs via cells called antigen-presenting cells. In the lymph node, these cells present the antigen to other cells of the immune system responsible for making antibodies and creating immunologic memory (see "How Do Vaccines Work?").

As a rule, a vaccine stimulates an immune response in the area where the vaccine is given, not throughout the body. Adjuvants, which are substances occasionally added to vaccines to enhance the immune response, also act only locally (see "Do Vaccines Contain Harmful Adjuvants Like Aluminum?"). All of this means that, for the most part, how much someone weighs doesn't matter because vaccines aren't distributed throughout the body.

The next logical question is, How are children protected against infections that enter through other places, like the nose, throat, or intestines? The answer is that although immune cells, like those that make antibodies, are typically generated where the vaccine is given, they travel throughout the body, offering protection at the many sites where infection might occur.

When vaccines are tested, dose-ranging studies are used. In this type of study, groups of participants are given different doses to determine which works best. The goal is to give the smallest amount of vaccine that can induce a protective immune response so that the vaccine is both effective and unlikely to cause side effects.

IS THERE ANY HARM IN USING AN ALTERNATIVE VACCINE SCHEDULE?

During the first few years of life, children may receive as many as twenty-seven separate inoculations and up to six shots at one time. For parents, it can be hard to watch their children restrained against their will and injected several times. Therefore, it's easy to see why some might prefer an alternative vaccine schedule that separates, delays, withholds, or spaces out vaccine doses.

The perceived value of an alternative schedule is that it might avoid weakening, overwhelming, or altering the young child's immune system. However, abundant evidence shows that vaccines do not cause these untoward effects, so changing the schedule would not add value (see "Safety").

Another argument people use for spacing out vaccines is that they contain potentially harmful additives that might be toxic if too many vaccines are given at once. But again, the evidence does not support this fear so changing the schedule will not increase the safety of vaccines (see "Ingredients").

Yet another specious argument is that getting too many vaccines is causing chronic conditions or diseases like asthma, allergies, autism, diabetes, and multiple sclerosis—which presumably could be avoided by choosing a different schedule. But again, no evidence supports these contentions of causality, so changing the schedule does not offer an advantage (see "Safety").

Some parents (and some doctors) argue that even if it's true that children's immune systems can easily handle the challenge of vaccines, there's no harm in spacing them out. However, there are several reasons that this is not true.

More Time Being Susceptible to Disease

The biggest problem with an alternative vaccine schedule is that it increases the time during which children are susceptible to vaccine-preventable diseases. If immunization rates across the United States were about 95 percent, this wouldn't be a problem.

Parents could hide their children within a highly protected population knowing they wouldn't be hurt by bacteria and viruses. But that's not the case. Herd (or community) immunity—the ability of a vaccinated community to protect those who can't or won't be vaccinated—has broken down. Consequently, outbreaks of pertussis are common; a measles epidemic in 2019 was larger than any year since the early 1990s; and children are starting to die from bacterial meningitis again because their parents are choosing either to delay or withhold vaccines. (For example, outbreaks of Hib meningitis caused the deaths of four unvaccinated children in Minnesota and Pennsylvania in 2008 and 2009.) Parents who choose to delay vaccines are taking an unnecessary risk without deriving any benefit.

No Data to Support the Safety or Effectiveness of an Alternative Vaccine Schedule

Another problem with alternative vaccine schedules is that they're untested. Every time a new vaccine is added to the recommended schedule, it's tested to make sure that it doesn't interfere with the immune response or safety of the existing vaccines or vice versa (see "How Do We Know That Different Vaccines Can Be Given at the Same Time?"). Making up a schedule that is untested takes an unnecessary risk, again without benefit. The irony of an alternative schedule is obvious: parents who opt out of the recommended schedule because of unfounded safety concerns are trading a schedule based on published studies in millions of children for one that has been formally tested in no children.

More Visits to the Doctor

Another reasonable-sounding argument for spacing out vaccines is that it would mean fewer shots at one time and therefore less pain for the child. However, researchers have found that children experience similar amounts of stress—as measured by the level of a hormone called cortisol—whether they are getting one shot or two at the same visit. This finding suggests that although children are clearly stressed by receiving a shot, two shots aren't more stressful than one. For this reason, separating or spacing out vaccinations, thus requiring more doctor's visits, would likely *increase* children's stress, could increase the risk of vaccination errors and missed vaccinations, and could result in greater out-of-pocket expenses for doctor's visits.

References

Offit, Paul A., and Charlotte A. Moser. "The Problem with Dr Bob's Alternative Vaccine Schedule." *Pediatrics* 123, no. 1 (2009): e164–69.

Ramsay, Douglas S., and Michael Lewis. "Developmental Changes in Infant Cortisol and Behavioral Response to Inoculation." *Child Development* 65, no. 5 (1994): 1491–1502.

WHY CAN'T VACCINES BE COMBINED TO REDUCE THE NUMBER OF SHOTS NEEDED?

Researchers have been combining vaccines for more than five decades. In the 1940s, they combined the diphtheria, tetanus, and pertussis vaccines into a single shot. Then, in the early 1970s, they combined the measles, mumps, and rubella vaccines into a single shot. Since then, combination vaccines have included measles, mumps, rubella, and chickenpox; *Haemophilus influenzae* type b (Hib) and hepatitis B; hepatitis A and hepatitis B; and diphtheria, tetanus, and pertussis added to various combinations of hepatitis B, polio, and Hib (see the section "Combination Vaccines"). Combination vaccines have reduced the number of shots that children get in the first few years of life, but not significantly since many vaccines require multiple doses.

So, why not make a single shot that combines all the vaccines? That way, children would need to get only one shot at two, four, six, and twelve to fifteen months of age and just one shot between four and six years of age. Unfortunately, combining vaccines is a lot harder than it sounds. Buffering agents (used to prolong shelf life) and stabilizing agents (used to distribute a vaccine evenly throughout the vial) for different vaccines may not be compatible when combined. Perhaps the best hope for relieving the burden of so many shots would be to start giving more vaccines by mouth or by skin patches. These technologies continue to be evaluated.

WHY AREN'T MORE VACCINES GIVEN BY MOUTH?

Of the more than a dozen vaccines given to children and adolescents, only one, the rotavirus vaccine, is given by mouth. Because this vaccine is designed to prevent an intestinal infection and because intestinal immunity is best induced by presenting vaccines to the intestinal surface, this makes sense.

But the intestines are loaded with immune cells perfectly capable of traveling throughout the body. So why not take advantage of the wealth of immune cells in the intestines and make a variety of oral vaccines? The answer is that we probably could. One obstacle is that the stomach makes a lot of acid and many proteases (enzymes that break down proteins) that can destroy certain vaccines. But technology is available to counter that, and it would be nice to see more vaccines given by mouth in the future.

CAN I AVOID THE NEED FOR VACCINES BY LIVING A HEALTHY LIFESTYLE?

Some people believe that living a healthy lifestyle—eating nutritious foods, getting plenty of exercise, and taking daily vitamins—is enough to avoid infections. Although good nutrition is important, immunity to specific viruses or bacteria can be acquired only by natural infection or immunization. And, as we know, the price of natural infection is often too high.

One example of why a healthy lifestyle doesn't provide enough protection can be found in the life of one of America's most beloved presidents, Franklin Delano Roosevelt. Roosevelt was an active, vigorous man. Coming from a wealthy family, he was certainly well nourished. But in his late thirties he contracted polio, a disease that permanently paralyzed him. Roosevelt died ten years (to the day) before the polio vaccine was first licensed in the United States—a vaccine that would have been the only reliable way for him to have avoided a disease from which he suffered for most of his life.

WHY SHOULD I TRUST A SYSTEM THAT MAKES MONEY FOR DRUG COMPANIES?

The pharmaceutical industry doesn't have a very good reputation. Indeed, the term "Big Pharma" is meant to be derogatory. And to some extent, the reputation is deserved. In marketing their products, pharmaceutical companies have acted aggressively, unethically, and sometimes illegally.

However, vaccines are not drugs. They're made differently, tested differently, regulated differently, promoted differently, and used differently.

First, vaccines are not nearly the moneymaker drugs are. Whereas cholesterol-lowering medications, hair loss and potency products, diabetes drugs, and anti-depressants are often used daily, vaccines are given only once or at most a few times during a person's life. For example, annual sales from a single cholesterol-lowering drug can exceed those for the entire worldwide vaccine industry. The pressure to sell drugs, which can be huge blockbusters for pharmaceutical companies, is great. With the possible exception of COVID-19 vaccines, however, there is no such thing as a blockbuster vaccine.

Second, vaccines are subjected to higher regulatory standards than drugs. Before drugs are licensed by the FDA, they are typically tested in hundreds or a few thousand people. Vaccines, on the other hand, are tested in tens of thousands of people:

- The pneumococcal vaccine, licensed in 2000, was tested in forty thousand children.
- The HPV vaccine, first licensed in 2006, was tested in thirty thousand women.

- Two rotavirus vaccines, licensed in 2006 and 2008, were tested in more than 130,000 children.
- The COVID-19 vaccines, authorized in 2020, were tested in more than seventy thousand people. '

Third, pharmaceutical companies don't have to convince people about the value of vaccines. That's because the groups that recommend vaccines—like the CDC and the AAP—do it for them. Recommending vaccines for routine use and publishing those recommendations in professional journals ensures that vaccines are a standard part of health care. The marketing dollars spent on vaccines are trivial compared to those spent on drugs.

A concern that vaccines can't be trusted because pharmaceutical companies have misrepresented or falsified their data would be justified if there were at least one example of this happening. But there isn't. Safety and efficacy data generated before licensure is invariably repeated in testing after licensure. And although some vaccines have been found to cause rare severe problems after licensure, it wasn't because the pharmaceutical companies had hidden or misrepresented data to the FDA before licensure; it was because the problem was too rare to have been picked up in prelicensure studies. For example, in the case of the rotavirus vaccine, a rare adverse event was found only after about one million children had been vaccinated (see the story of the RotaShield vaccine in "What Systems Are in Place to Ensure That Vaccines Are Safe?"). In this instance, the problem was quickly identified by post-licensure safety monitoring systems put in place by the CDC.

In summary, pharmaceutical companies that make vaccines should be trusted because they have an excellent record of making safe and effective products; because they have never been shown to knowingly misrepresent vaccine data in medical or scientific journals; because all study results, positive and negative, must be presented to the FDA before licensure; and because the vaccine-related efforts at pharmaceutical companies are often staffed by people with a background in public health interest in disease prevention. Although this might sound Pollyannaish, it's true.

SHOULD VACCINES BE MANDATED?

In a perfect world, vaccines wouldn't be mandated. People would be compelled by science-based information showing that the benefits of vaccines outweigh their risks. But we don't live in that world. Rather, we live in one where television shows, magazines, newspapers, and social media often present stories about vaccine risks that are untrue: that vaccines cause autism, diabetes, multiple sclerosis, learning disorders, chronic fatigue syndrome, and hyperactivity, among other problems. Consequently, some people, influenced by these stories, choose not to vaccinate themselves or their families.

To protect the population, we have vaccine mandates for admission to day care centers, schools, and even some workplaces. In the early 1900s, mandates were strictly enforced—there were no exceptions. But a series of court rulings in the late 1960s and early 1970s allowed parents to exempt their children from vaccination based on their religious beliefs. As of August 2023, forty-four states and the District of Columbia allowed such religious exemptions. It wasn't long before the courts also supported parents whose philosophical or personal beliefs precluded vaccination. By August 2023, twenty states allowed some type of philosophical exemptions. (For the latest information about exemptions by state, visit the website of Immunize.org: https://www.immunize.org/laws/exemptions.asp.)

One could reasonably argue that exemptions to vaccine mandates are a necessary concession when trying to compel an entire population to receive multiple vaccines during the first few years of life and that without exemptions, the number of people choosing not to get vaccines might only increase. But there's a problem with vaccine exemptions. And it's an obvious one.

Four studies have compared the incidence of measles and pertussis in states or localities that have high rates of vaccine exemptions—either philosophical or religious—with states or localities that have lower exemption rates. Unsurprisingly, areas with higher exemption rates have a higher incidence of vaccine-preventable infections. And as the number of vaccine exemptions continues to rise, the number of outbreaks of preventable infections will also rise. Eventually we may again have to ask ourselves whether mandates should be more strictly enforced—whether we can afford individual freedoms when they negatively affect the health of society.

References

Feiken, Daniel R., Dennis C. Lezotte, Richard F. Hamman, et al. "Individual and Community Risks of Measles and Pertussis Associated with Personal Exemptions to Immunization." *Journal of the American Medical Association* 284, no. 24 (2000): 3145–50.

Glanz, Jason M., David L. McClure, David J. Magid, et al. "Parental Refusal of Pertussis Vaccination Is Associated with an Increased Risk of Pertussis Infection in Children." *Pediatrics* 123, no. 6 (2009): 1446–51.

Omer, Saad B., William K. Y. Pan, Neal A. Halsey, et al. "Nonmedical Exemptions to School Immunization Requirements: Secular Trends and Association of State Policies with Pertussis Incidence." *Journal of the American Medical Association* 296, no. 14 (2006): 1757–63.

Salmon, Daniel A., Michael Haber, Eugene J. Gangarosa, et al. "Health Consequences of Religious and Philosophical Exemptions from Immunization Laws: Individual and Societal Risk of Measles." *Journal of the American Medical Association* 282, no. 1 (1999): 47–53.

IS IT MY SOCIAL RESPONSIBILITY TO GET VACCINATED?

The easiest way to answer this question is to look at health care providers who are asked to get vaccinated. In 2009, several U.S. hospitals required doctors, nurses, nurse practitioners, and others involved in patient care to receive an influenza vaccine. Certain facts were undeniable: (1) people made ill by the influenza virus are hospitalized every winter; (2) health care providers may catch influenza and inadvertently transmit it to those in their care; (3) people who come into the hospital with chronic lung, heart, or kidney disease are more likely to get severe and occasionally fatal influenza pneumonia; and (4) hospitals with more employees vaccinated against influenza have lower rates of virus transmission. Hospital officials mandated influenza vaccination out of concern for patient safety. The hospitals viewed health care providers as having not only a social responsibility but also a professional responsibility to protect their patients.

What about people who don't work in hospitals? Again, the facts are undeniable: people in states and regions with lower vaccination rates are more likely to suffer diseases like pertussis and measles (see "Should Vaccines Be Mandated?"). This was exemplified in the case, discussed earlier, of the unvaccinated boy from San Diego who caught measles in Switzerland and subsequently infected many others at home, including children too young to have been vaccinated (see "Why Do We Still Need Vaccines?"). The decision not to vaccinate affects not only that individual but also many others.

Some people who choose not to vaccinate will argue that if others are scared of catching vaccine-preventable infections, they can simply choose vaccination. But there are two problems with this thinking.

First, no vaccine is 100 percent effective; even those who are vaccinated can occasionally suffer severe infections. Further, as more and more people remain unvaccinated, the likelihood of disease in the community increases. Vaccinated and unvaccinated community members will be more likely to come into contact with someone who is infected. An outbreak of measles in the Netherlands in 1999 and 2000 is particularly instructive. It was found that children who were unvaccinated but living in a community with a high vaccination rate were much better off than those who were vaccinated but living in a community with a low vaccination rate.

Second, some people can't be vaccinated for medical reasons. These people might be receiving long-term steroids for rheumatological diseases (like lupus), chemotherapy for cancer, or immunosuppressive therapy for organ transplants, all of which alter a person's capacity to develop an effective immune response to vaccines. And some children are too young to receive certain vaccines. These people depend on a highly vaccinated community to protect them; if their community does not protect them, they're the ones most likely to suffer and die from vaccine-preventable infections. The ability of a vaccinated community to protect those who can't be vaccinated is called herd immunity. The percentage of vaccinated people necessary to provide herd immunity depends on the contagiousness of the virus or bacterium. For highly contagious infections, like measles, chickenpox, and pertussis, about 95 percent of the population must be immunized to prevent the spread of disease.

Some parents are starting to become concerned that the decisions of others are putting their children at risk; they worry that doctors' waiting rooms, places of worship, or classrooms with a high percentage of unvaccinated children have become dangerous. The clash between parents who exercise their right to leave their children unvaccinated and those who feel that this choice violates a social contract is growing. If outbreaks of vaccine-preventable infections continue, this conflict will only worsen.

References

Feiken, Daniel R., Dennis C. Lezotte, Richard F. Hamman, et al. "Individual and Community Risks of Measles and Pertussis Associated with Personal Exemptions to Immunization." *Journal of the American Medical Association* 284, no. 24 (2000): 3145–50.

Fine, Paul E. M., and Kim Mulholland. "Community Protection." In *Plotkin's Vaccines*, 8th ed., ed. Walter A. Orenstein, Paul A. Offit, Kathryn M. Edwards, and Stanley A. Plotkin. London: Elsevier, 2024: 1603–24.

Glanz, Jason M., David L. McClure, David J. Magid, et al. "Parental Refusal of Pertussis Vaccination Is Associated with an Increased Risk of Pertussis Infection in Children." *Pediatrics* 123, no. 6 (2009): 1446–51.

Offit, Paul A. "Fatal Exemption." *Wall Street Journal*, January 20, 2007.

Omer, Saad B., William K. Y. Pan, Neal A. Halsey, et al. "Nonmedical Exemptions to School Immunization Requirements: Secular Trends and Association of State Policies with Pertussis Incidence." *Journal of the American Medical Association* 296, no. 14 (2006): 1757–63.

Salmon, Daniel A., Michael Haber, Eugene J. Gangarosa, et al. "Health Consequences of Religious and Philosophical Exemptions from Immunization Laws: Individual and Societal Risk of Measles." *Journal of the American Medical Association* 282, no. 1 (1999): 47–53.

Van den Hof, Susan, Marina A. E. Conyn-van Spaendonck, and Jim E. van Steenbergen. "Measles Epidemic in the Netherlands, 1999–2000." *Journal of Infectious Diseases* 186, no. 10 (2002): 1483–86.

SAFETY

ARE VACCINES SAFE?

A vaccine is safe if its benefits definitively outweigh its risks. But any medical product that has a positive effect—whether a drug or a vaccine—can also have a negative effect. No vaccine is absolutely safe. All vaccines given as shots can cause pain, redness, or tenderness at the site of injection. And some vaccines can cause more serious problems. For example, the measles vaccine can cause a temporary decrease in platelets, which help the blood to clot. This happens in about one out of twenty-five thousand children who get the vaccine. This reaction, called thrombocytopenia, shouldn't be surprising since natural measles infection can do the same thing, except much more commonly and much more severely.

Other vaccine side effects can be quite severe. The chickenpox vaccine contains gelatin as a stabilizer. Some people are severely allergic to gelatin and can develop life-threatening allergic symptoms if they are given the chickenpox vaccine. The oral polio vaccine, no longer used in the United States but still in use in other parts of the world, can cause polio. It's rare, occurring in about one per 3.4 million doses, but it does happen. An influenza vaccine used in Europe during the swine flu pandemic in 2009 called Pandemrix was a rare cause of narcolepsy, a permanent disorder of wakefulness. And the yellow fever vaccine can be a rare cause of symptoms like yellow fever in older people.

But while there are rare risks to vaccines, nothing is risk free. The most dangerous aspect of vaccines is likely driving to the doctor's office to get them. Every year about forty thousand people in the United States die in car accidents. Walking outside on a rainy day isn't entirely safe; every year in the United States about thirty people are struck by lightning and killed. And tens of thousands of people die every year when they slip and fall. Even routine daily activities pose a certain degree of risk. But we choose to do them because we consider the benefits to outweigh the risks.

In the chapters that follow, we will describe in detail the benefits and risks of every vaccine. And you'll see that for people who don't have a preexisting medical condition or other reason that would preclude getting a vaccine, the benefits of every vaccine outweigh its risks.

HOW DO I KNOW IF A PROBLEM IS CAUSED BY A VACCINE?

Because we're human, we naturally look for reasons something happened. The process of seeking to understand what causes various problems has been crucial to our success as a species. And sometimes bad things happen, including to young children. They suffer asthma, allergies, autism, developmental delays, hyperactivity, or attention deficits, among other health problems. Worse: sometimes they die of poorly defined disorders, like sudden infant death syndrome (SIDS). Because children receive numerous vaccines during the first few years of life, some of these health conditions are diagnosed soon or immediately after receiving vaccines.

How can you know whether symptoms that follow a vaccination were caused by the vaccine? The best way is by performing scientific studies that compare a group of vaccinated individuals with a group of unvaccinated individuals who are otherwise similar. For example, in 1998, a British research group proposed that the combination measles-mumps-rubella (MMR) vaccine might cause autism. At the time, about one in two thousand children in England were diagnosed with autism, and about nine of ten were given the MMR vaccine. To determine whether the British research group's theory that the MMR vaccine caused autism was correct, researchers from around the world studied hundreds of thousands of children who did and did not receive the vaccine. If the vaccine caused autism, then the number of children with autism should be higher in the group that received the vaccine than in the group that didn't. As it turned out, the incidence of autism in children who got the MMR vaccine was the same as in those who didn't get it. (See "Do Vaccines Cause Autism?").

Importantly, when trying to determine whether a vaccine causes a particular problem, one study isn't enough; other investigators should repeat it to make sure that the results hold up across different populations of children. That was done with investigations into the MMR-causes-autism theory. Eighteen studies performed by researchers in seven countries on three continents costing tens of millions of dollars all showed the same thing: the MMR vaccine didn't cause autism. Although epidemiological studies looking at disease rates among populations are not perfect, they can be quite powerful, particularly when numerous studies by different researchers taking somewhat different experimental approaches find the same thing. Indeed, epidemiological studies can determine whether a vaccine caused a problem in as few as one in a million vaccinated children.

Many parents who read about the investigations into the MMR vaccine were reassured by the results, but some weren't. They had been compelled by individual anecdotes they had witnessed or heard about, and no study could convince them otherwise.

ONE PERSON'S STORY

Anecdotal experiences can be powerful. For example, a professor emeritus at the Duke University School of Medicine told the
story of a friend's four-month-old infant who had been taken to
a clinic to get the diphtheria, tetanus, and pertussis (DTaP) vaccine. The father waited and waited in line. Finally, he grew tired
and took his baby home *without* getting the vaccine. At home, he
put the child to bed. Several hours later, the child was found dead
in his crib, a victim of sudden infant death syndrome (SIDS).
Had the child received the vaccine, no amount of statistical evidence in the world would likely have convinced this father that
anything other than the vaccine was the cause.

Source: Sam Katz communication with author (2000).

Reference

Myers, Martin G., and Diego Pineda. *Do Vaccines Cause That?! A Guide
    for Evaluating Vaccine Safety Concerns*. Galveston, TX: Immuniza-
    tions for Public Health, 2008.

WHAT SYSTEMS ARE IN PLACE TO ENSURE THAT VACCINES ARE SAFE?

Before they're licensed, vaccines are tested in tens of thousands
of children. These studies are large enough to determine whether
vaccines cause common or even uncommon side effects, but
they are not large enough to determine whether a vaccine may
cause a very rare side effect. To monitor instances of very rare
side effects, two post-licensure systems were put in place in the
late 1980s and early 1990s: the Vaccine Adverse Event Reporting
System (VAERS) and the Vaccine Safety Datalink (VSD).

VAERS is a surveillance system codirected by the Food and
Drug Administration (FDA) and the Centers for Disease Control and Prevention (CDC). If a parent, health care provider, or

anyone else believes that a vaccine has caused an adverse event (i.e., a harmful or unwanted side effect), they can complete and submit a one-page form. These forms—which are easily obtained from doctors' offices or from the internet (http://vaers.hhs.gov /index)—are carefully evaluated by the FDA and the CDC to determine whether a particular side effect is reported more frequently than would be expected.

One example of how VAERS works occurred between 1998 and 1999 when a new vaccine to prevent rotavirus, RotaShield, was licensed by the FDA and recommended for routine use in children to be given by mouth at two, four, and six months of age. Soon after the vaccine was introduced, reports of an unusual problem, an intestinal blockage called intussusception, started coming into VAERS. Intussusception is a medical emergency that occurs when one part of the intestine telescopes into another, causing a blockage. When this happens, the blood supply to the intestinal surface can be compromised, and the intestinal lining can become severely damaged. Without medical treatment, children can suffer massive intestinal bleeding. Also, bacteria that normally live on the intestinal surface can enter the bloodstream, causing a serious infection. Either of these problems can be fatal.

After RotaShield had been given for several months, fifteen cases of intussusception were reported to VAERS. This was more than had been reported for any previous vaccine. Although it was tempting at this point to conclude that RotaShield caused intussusception, VAERS data alone were not adequate to prove this. Investigators now had to determine whether intussusception following RotaShield administration was occurring at a rate greater than would be expected by chance alone (before this vaccine was first used, intussusception occurred in about one out of every two thousand infants annually). To do this, they used the VSD.

The VSD is a group of large health maintenance organizations whose computerized medical records are linked, representing about 3 percent of the U.S. population, including both adults and children. Whereas VAERS can be used to generate a hypothesis (e.g., whether a vaccine has caused a particular problem), the VSD can be used to answer the question because it offers something that VAERS doesn't: a control group. In the case of the rotavirus vaccine, investigators could examine the medical records of children who either had or had not received RotaShield to see whether intussusception occurred more commonly in the vaccinated group. It did. RotaShield caused intussusception in about one in every ten thousand children who got the vaccine. Consequently, RotaShield was taken off the market. This was the first time a vaccine had been discontinued because of a safety problem in almost fifty years.

Seven years passed before another rotavirus vaccine was given to U.S. children. It was called RotaTeq, and it was made differently from RotaShield in that it was based on rotaviruses that infect cows rather than monkeys. This time, the VSD was immediately put into action using something called rapid-cycle analysis. As soon as children started to receive RotaTeq, VSD investigators began examining the incidence of intussusception in children who either had or had not received it. They evaluated these children's records *every day*, looking for any evidence that RotaTeq was causing the same problem as RotaShield. But the incidence of intussusception was the same in both groups of children.

Another example of the use of VAERS and the VSD is myocarditis (an inflammation of the heart) following receipt of mRNA vaccines to prevent COVID-19. Following the authorization of two mRNA vaccines in December 2020, reports to VAERS of myocarditis triggered studies in the VSD that found the association was real, not just a coincidence. However, while myocarditis occurs rarely after receipt of an mRNA COVID-19 vaccine (about one case per fifty thousand doses), it occurs far more commonly following natural COVID-19 infection (about one case per one hundred infections).

VAERS and the VSD are model systems to determine whether a vaccine causes a very rare side effect. They've served us well, showing that vaccines don't cause diseases or conditions like multiple sclerosis, allergies, asthma, or diabetes, among others.

References

Centers for Disease Control and Prevention. "Clinical Considerations: Myocarditis and Pericarditis After Receipt of COVID-19 Vaccines Among Adolescents and Young Adults." Last reviewed October 10, 2023. http://www.cdc.gov/vaccines/covid-19/clinical-considerations/myocarditis.html.

Centers for Disease Control and Prevention. "Postmarketing Monitoring of Intussusception After RotaTeq Vaccination—United States, February 1, 2006–February 15, 2007." *Morbidity and Mortality Weekly Report* 56, no. 10 (2007): 218–22.

Kramarz, Piotr, Eric K. France, Frank DeStefano, et al. "Population-Based Study of Rotavirus Vaccination and Intussusception." *Pediatric Infectious Diseases Journal* 20, no. 4 (2001): 410–16.

Murphy, Trudy V., Paul M. Gargiullo, Mehran S. Massoudi, et al. "Intussusception Among Infants Given an Oral Rotavirus Vaccine." *New England Journal of Medicine* 344, no. 8 (2001): 564–72.

DO VACCINES CAUSE CHRONIC DISEASES?

Although vaccines have clearly extended our lives, some people fear that vaccines have merely substituted chronic diseases for infectious diseases. These people believe that instead of suffering from measles, mumps, and chickenpox, we now suffer from diabetes, multiple sclerosis, and arthritis, all of which are autoimmune conditions (in which the body reacts against itself).

It is certainly true that some infections can cause the body to react against itself. One example is strep throat, which is caused by the bacterium *Streptococcus pyogenes*. Some children infected with strep develop a disease that can severely affect the heart. This happens because proteins on the surface of strep bacteria (called M proteins) are very similar to proteins found on the cells that line the heart. When the immune system reacts to strep bacteria, it also inadvertently reacts to the heart. The result is a severe and occasionally fatal disease: rheumatic fever.

Another example is Lyme disease, caused by the bacterium *Borrelia burgdorferi*. People with Lyme disease develop a long-lived, recurrent arthritis because one of the Lyme bacterial proteins is like a protein found in joints. And intestinal infections caused by *Campylobacter* bacteria can lead to an autoimmune disease called Guillain-Barré syndrome (GBS), which causes the body to attack lining of nerves.

If infections can cause the body to react against itself, it stands to reason that vaccines could do the same thing. But vaccines don't have what it takes to cause the autoimmunity occasionally found after natural infection. For example, multiple sclerosis is an autoimmune disease of the brain in which the body reacts against the covering of nerves. Nerves are like wires covered by a thin layer of rubber. But instead of rubber, nerves are covered by something called myelin, the principal component of which is myelin basic protein. The symptoms experienced by people with multiple sclerosis are often worse during the winter. That's because influenza infections occur most commonly during the winter, and one of the proteins on influenza virus can mimic myelin basic protein. Thus, the bodies of some people with multiple sclerosis, when making an immune response against influenza virus, also inadvertently make an immune response to their own brain. Knowing this, a logical next question is, Can influenza vaccine do what natural influenza infections do? The influenza vaccine is like a natural influenza virus in that both contain the protein that mimics myelin basic protein. But studies have clearly shown that although natural infection can worsen multiple sclerosis symptoms, the influenza vaccine can't. That's because the influenza vaccine virus doesn't reproduce (it's not live) and therefore doesn't induce nearly the intensity of the immune response necessary to cause the body to react against itself. (Even the nasal-spray influenza vaccine, which is live and can reproduce, doesn't reproduce very well, so, like the killed influenza vaccine, it doesn't cause the body to react against itself either.)

Lyme disease is another example of why vaccines don't induce very good autoimmune responses. As mentioned, Lyme disease can cause a type of chronic arthritis based on an autoimmune response to a surface protein on the bacteria that is similar to a protein found in joints. This bacterial surface protein was used to make a Lyme disease vaccine that was available in the United States between 1998 and 2002. The obvious question is, Did the Lyme disease vaccine cause chronic arthritis? To answer this question, tens of thousands of people who had received the vaccine were compared with tens of thousands of people who didn't to see whether the risk of arthritis was greater in the vaccinated group. It wasn't. Unfortunately, however, because of unfounded safety concerns, the vaccine was not well accepted, and the company stopped making it. This is an example of an existing technology that could prevent illness and suffering but instead sits on a shelf simply because misinformation won the day.

Vaccines have demonstrated that they can't cause the cascade of immunological events necessary for autoimmunity. They have consistently been shown not to cause multiple sclerosis, diabetes, or other autoimmune diseases. Historically, one exception to this rule was the swine flu vaccine given to prevent a feared influenza pandemic in 1976, which was found to be a rare cause of Guillain-Barré syndrome in about one out of one hundred thousand vaccine recipients. Another exception to the rule was an influenza vaccine used in Europe in 2009 (Pandemrix), which was found to be a rare cause of narcolepsy, a permanent disorder of wakefulness.

References

GENERAL

Offit, Paul A., and Charles J. Hackett. "Addressing Parents' Concerns: Do Vaccines Cause Allergic or Autoimmune Diseases?" *Pediatrics* 111, no. 3 (2003): 653–59.

INFLUENZA VACCINE STUDIES

De Keyser, Jacques, Cornelis Zwanikken, and Maartje Boon. "Effects of Influenza Vaccination and Influenza Illness on Exacerbations in Multiple Sclerosis." *Journal of Neurological Sciences* 159, no. 1 (1998): 51–53.

Miller, A. E., L. A. Morgante, L. Y. Buchwald, et al. "A Multicenter, Randomized, Double-Blind, Placebo-Controlled Trial of Influenza Immunization in Multiple Sclerosis." *Neurology* 48, no. 2 (1997): 312–14.

Moriabadi, N. F., S. Niewiesk, N. Kruse, et al. "Influenza Vaccination in MS: Absence of T-Cell Response Against White Matter Proteins." *Neurology* 56, no. 7 (2001): 938–43.

Schonberger, Lawrence B. Dennis J. Bregman, John Z. Sullivan-Bolyai, et al. "Guillain-Barré Syndrome Following Vaccination in the National Immunization Program, United States, 1976–1977," *American Journal of Epidemiology* 110, no. 2 (1979) 105–23.

LYME DISEASE VACCINE STUDIES

Lathrop, Sarah L., Robert Ball, Penina Haber, et al. "Adverse Event Reports Following Vaccination for Lyme Disease: December 1998–July 2000." *Vaccine* 20, nos. 11–12 (2002): 1603–8.

Sigal, Leonard H., John M. Zahradnik, Philip Lavin, et al. "A Vaccine Consisting of Recombinant *Borrelia Burgdorferi* Outer-Surface Protein A to Prevent Lyme Disease." *New England Journal of Medicine* 339, no. 4 (1998): 216–22.

Steere, Allen C., Vijay K. Sikand, François Meurice, et al. "Vaccination Against Lyme Disease with Recombinant *Borrelia Burgdorferi* Outer-Surface Lipoprotein A with Adjuvant." *New England Journal of Medicine* 339, no. 4 (1998): 209–15.

DO VACCINES CAUSE AUTISM?

The notion that vaccines cause autism was launched on February 28, 1998. That's when researchers in England published a paper claiming that the combination measles-mumps-rubella (MMR) vaccine caused autism. The British group suggested that the measles vaccine damaged the intestine, allowing brain-damaging proteins to escape the gut and enter the brain. Other scientists tried to find the same results but couldn't: no intestinal inflammation, no brain-damaging proteins, and no clear route to the brain. The paper was later retracted, meaning it was removed from the publication, after it became apparent that the lead author, Dr. Andrew Wakefield, had been untruthful about his funding, potential conflicts of interest, and some of the report's findings. More importantly, however, eighteen subsequent studies found no evidence that children who receive the MMR vaccine are at greater risk of autism than those who don't.

In 1999, the hypothesis shifted. At that time, the American Academy of Pediatrics, together with the U.S. Public Health Service, asked for thimerosal, an ethylmercury-containing preservative, to be removed from all vaccines given to young children. These groups had become concerned that as more and more vaccines containing thimerosal were added to the schedule, babies might be exposed to harmful quantities of mercury. Those in favor of removing thimerosal argued that they were exercising caution in the absence of data because at the time, no studies had determined that the overall quantity of thimerosal received across multiple vaccines was toxic. Unfortunately, the decision to remove thimerosal was made so quickly that some parents became concerned. They reasoned that maybe thimerosal caused autism. As had been the case during the MMR scare, the science quickly followed. Six studies examined the risk of autism in those who either had or had not received vaccines containing thimerosal, and all showed that the chance of getting autism was the same in both groups. Consistent with these findings, the incidence of autism has only continued to increase even though thimerosal has been removed from all vaccines given to young infants. Three other studies found that thimerosal in vaccines didn't cause even subtle signs of mercury poisoning.

A few years later, the hypothesis shifted again. This time some parents feared that autism was caused by too many vaccines given too early. Another study was done comparing the rates of autism and other neurodevelopmental or psychological disorders in children who were vaccinated according to the recommended schedule with the rates in children whose parents had chosen to delay or withhold vaccines. Again, no difference was found between the two groups. Delaying or withholding vaccines didn't reduce the risk of autism. It only increased the risk of getting vaccine-preventable diseases.

Coincident with the studies related to vaccines and autism, other researchers were working to identify the causes of autism. While we still do not understand all the reasons that some children develop autism, we have continued to learn more. For example, we know that both genes and environmental conditions, particularly during fetal development, can play a role. Exposure to medications, such as thalidomide, or viral infections, like rubella, during pregnancy can cause an infant to have autism. Parental age, particularly that of the father, has also been found to play a role.

For the latest science on autism and for support resources and research studies for families affected by this increasingly common condition, visit the Autism Science Foundation website: https://www.autismsciencefoundation.org.

References

MMR VACCINE

Afzal, M. A., L. C. Ozoemena, A. O'Hare, et al. "Absence of Detectable Measles Virus Genome Sequence in Blood of Autistic Children Who Have Had Their MMR Vaccination During the Routine Childhood Immunization Schedule of UK." *Journal of Medical Virology* 78, no. 5 (2006): 623–30.

Dales, Loring, Sandra Jo Hammer, and Natalie J. Smith. "Time Trends in Autism and in MMR Immunization Coverage in California." *Journal of the American Medical Association* 285, no. 9 (2001): 1183–85.

Davis, Robert L., Piotr Kramarz, Kari Bohlke, et al. "Measles-Mumps-Rubella and Other Measles-Containing Vaccines Do

Not Increase the Risk for Inflammatory Bowel Disease: A Case-Control Study from the Vaccine Safety Datalink Project." *Archives of Pediatrics and Adolescent Medicine* 155, no. 3 (2002): 354–59.

DeStefano, Frank, Tanya K. Bhasin, William W. Thompson, et al. "Age at First Measles-Mumps-Rubella Vaccination in Children with Autism and School-Matched Control Subjects: A Population-Based Study in Metropolitan Atlanta." *Pediatrics* 113, no. 2 (2004): 259–66.

DeStefano, Frank, and Robert T. Chen. "Negative Association Between MMR and Autism." *Lancet* 353, no. 9169 (1999): 1986–87.

D'Souza, Yasmin, Eric Fombonne, and Brian J. Ward. "No Evidence of Persisting Measles Virus in Peripheral Blood Mononuclear Cells from Children with Autism Spectrum Disorder." *Pediatrics* 118, no. 4 (2006): 1664–75.

Farrington, C. Paddy, Elizabeth Miller, and Brent Taylor. "MMR and Autism: Further Evidence Against a Causal Association." *Vaccine* 19, no. 27 (2001): 3632–35.

Fombonne, Eric. "Are Measles Infections or Measles Immunizations Linked to Autism?" *Journal of Autism and Developmental Disorders* 29, no. 4 (1999): 349–50.

Fombonne, Eric, and Suniti Chakrabarti. "No Evidence for a New Variant of Measles-Mumps-Rubella-Induced Autism." *Pediatrics* 108, no. 4 (2001): e58.

Fombonne, Eric, and E. H. Cook Jr. "MMR and Autistic Enterocolitis: Consistent Epidemiological Failure to Find an Association." *Molecular Psychiatry* 8, no. 2 (2003): 133–34.

Halsey, Neal A., and Susan L. Hyman. "Measles-Mumps-Rubella Vaccine and Autistic Spectrum Disorder: Report from the New Challenges in Childhood Immunization Conference Convened in Oak Brook, Illinois, June 12, 2000." *Pediatrics* 107, no. 5 (2001): e84.

Honda, Hideo, Yasuo Shimizu, and Michael Rutter. "No Effect of MMR Withdrawal on the Incidence of Autism: A Total Population Study." *Journal of Child Psychiatry and Psychology* 46, no. 6 (2005): 572–79.

Kaye, James A., Maria del Mar Melero-Montes, and Hershel Jick. "Measles, Mumps, and Rubella Vaccine and the Incidence of

Autism Recorded by General Practitioners: A Time Trend Analysis." *British Medical Journal* 322, no. 7284 (2001): 460–63.

Madsen, Kreesten M., Anders Hviid, Mogens Vestergaard, et al. "A Population-Based Study of Measles, Mumps, and Rubella Vaccination and Autism." *New England Journal of Medicine* 347, no. 19 (2002): 1477–82.

Mäkela, Annamari, J. Pekka Nuorti, and Heikki Peltola. "Neurologic Disorders After Measles-Mumps-Rubella Vaccination." *Pediatrics* 110, no. 5 (2002): 957–63.

Offit, Paul A., and Susan E. Coffin. "Communicating Science to the Public: MMR Vaccine and Autism." *Vaccine* 22, no. 1 (2003): 1–6.

Peltola, Heikki, Annamari Patja, Pauli Leinikki, et al. "No Evidence for Measles, Mumps, and Rubella Vaccine-Associated Inflammatory Bowel Disease or Autism in a 14-Year Prospective Study." *Lancet* 351, no. 9112 (1998): 1327–28.

Taylor, Brent, Elizabeth Miller, C. Paddy Farrington, et al. "Autism and Measles, Mumps, and Rubella Vaccine: No Epidemiological Evidence for a Causal Association." *Lancet* 353, no. 9169 (1999): 2026–29.

Taylor, Brent, Elizabeth Miller, Raghu Lingam, et al. "Measles, Mumps, and Rubella Vaccination and Bowel Problems or Developmental Regression in Children with Autism: Population Study." *British Medical Journal* 324, no. 7334 (2002): 393–96.

Wilson, Kumanan, Ed Mills, Cory Ross, et al. "Association of Autistic Spectrum Disorder and the Measles, Mumps, and Rubella Vaccine." *Archives of Pediatrics and Adolescent Medicine* 157, no. 7 (2003): 628–34.

THIMEROSAL

Andrews, Nick, Elizabeth Miller, Andrew Grant, et al. "Thimerosal Exposure in Infants and Developmental Disorders: A Retrospective Cohort Study in the United Kingdom Does Not Support a Causal Association." *Pediatrics* 114, no. 3 (2004): 584–91.

Fombonne, Eric, Rita Zakarian, Andrew Bennett, et al. "Pervasive Developmental Disorders in Montreal, Quebec, Canada: Prevalence and Links with Immunizations." *Pediatrics* 118, no. 1 (2006): e139–50.

Heron, Jon, and Jean Golding. "Thimerosal Exposure in Infants and Developmental Disorders: A Prospective Cohort Study in the United Kingdom Does Not Support a Causal Association." *Pediatrics* 114, no. 3 (2004): 577–83.

Hviid, Anders, Michael Stellfeld, Jan Wohlfahrt, and Mads Melbye. "Association Between Thimerosal-Containing Vaccine and Autism." *Journal of the American Medical Association* 290, no. 13 (2003): 1763–66.

Institute of Medicine. *Immunization Safety Review: Vaccines and Autism.* Washington, DC: National Academies Press, 2004.

Madsen, Kreesten M., Marlene B. Lauritsen, Carsten B. Pedersen, et al. "Thimerosal and the Occurrence of Autism: Negative Ecological Evidence from Danish Population-Based Data." *Pediatrics* 112, no. 3, pt. 1 (2003): 604–6.

Schechter, Robert, and Judith K. Grether. "Continuing Increases in Autism Reported to California's Development Services System: Mercury in Retrograde." *Archives of General Psychiatry* 65, no. 1 (2008): 19–24.

Stehr-Green, Paul, Peet Tull, Michael Stellfeld, et al. "Autism and Thimerosal-Containing Vaccines: Lack of Consistent Evidence for an Association." *American Journal of Preventive Medicine* 25, no. 2 (2005): 101–6.

Thompson, William W., Cristofer Price, Barbara Goodson, et al. "Early Thimerosal Exposure and Neuropsychological Outcomes at 7 to 10 Years." *New England Journal of Medicine* 357, no. 13 (2007): 1281–92.

TOO MANY VACCINES TOO EARLY

Smith, Michael J., and Charles R. Woods. "On-Time Vaccine Receipt in the First Year Does Not Adversely Affect Neuropsychological Outcomes." *Pediatrics* 125, no. 6 (2010): 1134–41.

DO VACCINES CAUSE ALLERGIES OR ASTHMA?

Several types of antibodies circulate in the body. One type, immunoglobulin G (IgG), is commonly found in the bloodstream. Another type, immunoglobulin A (IgA), is commonly found at the lining of the nose, throat, and intestines. But it's the third one, immunoglobulin E (IgE), that can be particularly troublesome because it mediates most allergic diseases, like hay fever and asthma. During an allergic response, IgE binds to a type of cell in the body called a mast cell. Mast cells release inflammation mediators (such as histamine) that cause wheezing, hives, sneezing, runny nose, and itchy eyes.

Several factors control IgE. The most important is a type of immune cell called T cells. The two most important types of T cells with regard to allergies and asthma are T-helper cell type 1 (Th1) and T-helper cell type 2 (Th2). Th1 cells decrease the production of IgE, and Th2 cells increase the production of IgE. So, when talking about allergies, Th1 cells are good, and Th2 cells are bad.

At birth, babies have a predominance of Th2 cells, which bias immune responses toward allergic responses. The best way to overcome this is to enhance the production of Th1 cells. This occurs naturally by infection with bacteria and viruses, both of which prompt the body to produce more Th1 cells. The most succinct description of this phenomenon and the importance of experiencing infections in the first few years of life can be found in the subtitle of an editorial in the *New England Journal of Medicine*: "Please, Sneeze on My Child."

Some people fear that because vaccines prevent natural infections, the maturation of Th1 cells might be affected, thus causing children to develop allergies or asthma (this is often referred to as the "hygiene hypothesis"). For example, children who live in large families, attend day care, or live in low- or middle-income countries—and are therefore exposed to more bacteria and viruses than other children—are less likely to have allergies than other children. So, the hygiene hypothesis makes sense. But for a couple of reasons, it doesn't extend to vaccines.

First, vaccines do not prevent most common childhood infections. For example, a study of twenty-five thousand illnesses in Cleveland in the 1960s found that children experienced six to eight infections a year in the first six years of life, most of which were viral infections of the upper respiratory tract or intestines that aren't prevented by vaccines. They were caused by viruses, such as parainfluenza virus, rhinovirus, respiratory syncytial virus (RSV), adenovirus, parechovirus, enterovirus, coxsackie virus, norovirus, calicivirus, and astrovirus. Therefore, vaccines are unlikely to prevent most common childhood infections and won't alter the normal balance of Th1 and Th2 cells.

Second, diseases prevented by vaccines, such as pertussis, measles, mumps, rubella, and chickenpox, are highly contagious and easily transmitted independent of the degree of hygiene in the home or the level of sanitation in the country. So, the hygiene hypothesis doesn't hold here.

Clinical studies also support the idea that vaccines don't cause allergies or asthma. One group of investigators examined computerized records of more than eighteen thousand children born between 1991 and 1997 who were enrolled in four large health maintenance organizations. Children who had received the diphtheria-pertussis-tetanus, oral polio, *Haemophilus influenzae* type b (Hib), hepatitis B, and MMR vaccines were found not to be at greater risk for asthma than those who hadn't. Another well-controlled study of more than six hundred children found that those who had received the diphtheria-tetanus-pertussis vaccine were not at greater risk for asthma, hives, or food allergies. Several other studies also found no evidence that vaccines increased the risk for allergic diseases.

Taken together, these studies show that vaccines do not cause allergies or asthma.

References

Anderson, H. Ross, Jan D. Poloniecki, David P. Strachan, et al. "Immunization and Symptoms of Atopic Disease in Children: Results from the International Study of Asthma and Allergies in Children." *American Journal of Public Health* 91, no. 7 (2001): 1126–29.

Ball, Thomas M., Jose A. Castro-Rodriguez, Kent A. Griffith, et al. "Siblings, Day-Care Attendance, and the Risk of Asthma and Wheezing During Childhood." *New England Journal of Medicine* 343, no. 8 (2000): 538–43.

Christiansen, Sandra C. "Day Care, Siblings, and Asthma—Please, Sneeze on My Child." *New England Journal of Medicine* 343, no. 8 (2000): 574–75.

DeStefano, Frank, David Gu, Piotr Kramarz, et al. "Childhood Vaccinations and Risk of Asthma." *Pediatric Infectious Disease Journal* 21, no. 6 (2002): 498–504.

Dingle, John H., George F. Badger, and William S. Jordan Jr. *Illness in the Home: A Study of 25,000 Illnesses in a Group of Cleveland Families.* Cleveland: Press of Western Reserve University, 1964.

Kay, A. B. "Allergy and Allergic Diseases." *New England Journal of Medicine* 344, no. 1 (2001): 30–37.

Kramarz, Piotr, Frank DeStefano, Paul M. Gargiullo, et al. "Does Influenza Vaccination Exacerbate Asthma? Analysis of a Large Cohort of Children with Asthma." *Archives of Family Medicine* 9, no. 7 (2000): 617–23.

Nilsson, L., N. Kjellman, and B. Bjorksten. "A Randomized Controlled Trial of the Effect of Pertussis Vaccines on Atopic Disease." *Archives of Pediatrics and Adolescent Medicine* 152, no. 8 (1998): 734–38.

Ponsonby, Anne-Louise, David Couper, Terence Dwyer, et al. "Relationship Between Early Life Respiratory Illness, Family Size Over Time, and the Development of Asthma and Hay Fever: A Seven-Year Follow-Up Study." *Thorax* 54, no. 8 (1999): 664–69.

Prescott, Susan L., Claudia Macaubas, Barbara J. Holt, et al. "Transplacental Priming of the Human Immune System to Environmental Allergens: Universal Skewing of Initial T Cell Responses Toward the Th2 Cytokine Profile." *Journal of Immunology* 160, no. 10 (1998): 4730–37.

Wills-Karp, Marsha, Joanna Santeliz, and Christopher L. Karp. "The Germless Theory of Allergic Disease: Revisiting the Hygiene Hypothesis." *Nature Reviews Immunology* 1, no. 1 (2001): 69–75.

DO VACCINES CAUSE CANCER?

In the 1950s and 1960s, scientists invented two polio vaccines. One, made by Jonas Salk, involved inactivating poliovirus with formaldehyde. The other, made by Albert Sabin, involved weakening poliovirus by growing it in nonhuman cells (see "How Are Vaccines Made?"). Both strategies shared an important feature: the vaccine viruses were grown in monkey kidney cells.

In 1960, another researcher, Bernice Eddy, found that monkey kidney cells used to make polio vaccines contained another virus: a monkey virus. Because it was the fortieth monkey virus identified, it was called simian virus 40 (SV40). This meant that children inoculated with Salk's and Sabin's vaccines had also been inadvertently inoculated with SV40 virus. This was a problem because Eddy later found that SV40 virus, when injected into newborn hamsters, caused large tumors to develop under the skin, as well as in the lungs, kidneys, and brain. At the time of this discovery, Salk's vaccine had already been injected into tens of millions of people, and thousands more were receiving it every day. Sabin's vaccine hadn't been licensed in the United States, but it had been given to ninety million people in Russia, mostly children.

During the next few years, researchers performed a series of studies that were reassuring. They found that although SV40 caused cancer when injected into hamsters, it didn't cause cancer when it was fed to them. Sabin's vaccine was swallowed, not injected. Researchers later found SV40 in the feces of children given Sabin's vaccine, but none of those children developed antibodies to the virus. Apparently, SV40 just passed through the intestines without causing an infection. Researchers also found that although the formaldehyde used in Salk's vaccine didn't completely kill SV40, it did decrease its infectivity by at least ten-thousand-fold. The quantity of residual SV40 virus in Salk's vaccine probably wasn't enough to cause cancer. But at that point, no one was sure.

Horrified that some children had been injected with a potentially cancer-causing virus, researchers compared cancer rates in children who had received a vaccine contaminated with SV40 to the rates in unvaccinated children. Eight years after the tainted vaccines had been given, the incidence of cancer was the same in both groups, and the same was true fifteen and thirty years later. And it was true for children who had received SV40-contaminated vaccines in the United States, the United Kingdom, Germany, and Sweden. By the mid-1990s, public health officials were confident that the inadvertent contamination of polio vaccines with SV40 didn't cause cancer.

No vaccines made today contain SV40 virus.

References

Carroll-Pankhurst, C., E. A. Engels, H. D. Strickler, et al. "Thirty-Five Year Mortality Following Receipt of SV40-Contaminated Polio Vaccine During the Neonatal Period." *British Journal of Cancer* 85, no. 9 (2001): 1295–97.

Engels, E. A., J. Chen, R. P. Viscidi, et al. "Poliovirus Vaccination During Pregnancy, Maternal Seroconversion to Simian Virus 40, and Risk of Childhood Cancer." *American Journal of Epidemiology* 160, no. 4 (2004): 306–16.

Engels, Eric A., Hormuzd A. Katki, Nété M. Nielson, et al. "Cancer Incidence in Denmark Following Exposure to Poliovirus Vaccine Contaminated with Simian Virus 40." *Journal of the National Cancer Institute* 95, no. 7 (2003): 532–39.

Engels, Eric A., Leonard H. Rodman, Morton Frisch, et al. "Childhood Exposure to Simian Virus 40-Contaminated Poliovirus Vaccine and Risk of AIDS-Associated Non-Hodgkin's Lymphoma." *International Journal of Cancer* 106, no. 2 (2003): 283–87.

Ferber, Dan. "Creeping Consensus on SV40 and Polio Vaccine." *Science* 298, no. 5594 (2002): 725–27.

Fraumeni, Joseph F., Jr., Charles R. Stark, Eli Gold, and Martha L. Lepow. "Simian Virus 40 in Polio Vaccine: Follow-Up of Newborn Recipients." *Science* 167, no. 3914 (1970): 59–60.

Innis, M. D. "Oncogenesis and Poliomyelitis Vaccine." *Nature* 219, no. 5157 (1968): 972–73.

Mortimer, Edward A., Martha L. Lepow, Eli Gold, et al. "Long-Term Follow-Up of Persons Inadvertently Inoculated with SV40 as Neonates." *New England Journal of Medicine* 305, no. 25 (1981): 1517–18.

Olin, P., and J. Giesecke. "Potential Exposure to SV40 in Polio Vaccines Used in Sweden During 1957: No Impact on Cancer Incidence Rates 1960 to 1993." *Development of Biological Standards* 94 (1998): 227–33.

Rollison, Dana E. M., William F. Page, Harriet Crawford, et al. "Case-Control Study of Cancer Among U.S. Army Veterans Exposed to Simian Virus 40-Contaminated Adenovirus Vaccine." *American Journal of Epidemiology* 160, no. 4 (2004): 317–24.

Shah, Keerti, and Neal Nathanson. "Human Exposure to SV40: Review and Comment." *American Journal of Epidemiology* 103, no. 1 (1976): 1–12.

Shah, Keerti V., Harvey L. Ozer, Harry S. Pond, et al. "SV40 Neutralizing Antibodies in Sera of U.S. Residents Without History of Polio Immunization." *Nature* 231, no. 5303 (1971): 448–49.

Stenton, S. C. "Simian Virus 40 and Human Malignancy." *British Medical Journal* 316, no. 7135 (1998): 877–80.

Strickler, H. D., and J. J. Goedert. "Exposure to SV40-Contaminated Poliovirus Vaccine and the Risk of Cancer: A Review of the Epidemiologic Evidence." *Development of Biological Standards* 94 (1998): 235–44.

Strickler, Howard D., Philip S. Rosenberg, Susan S. Devesa, et al. "Contamination of Poliovirus Vaccines with Simian Virus 40 (1955–1963) and Subsequent Cancer Rates." *Journal of the American Medical Association* 279, no. 4 (1998): 292–95.

Strickler, Howard D., Philip S. Rosenberg, Susan S. Devesa, et al. "Contamination of Poliovirus Vaccine with SV40 and the Incidence of Medulloblastoma." *Medical and Pediatric Oncology* 32, no. 1 (1999): 77–78.

Vilchez, Regis A., Amy S. Arrington, and Janet S. Butel. "Re: Cancer Incidence in Denmark Following Exposure to Poliovirus Vaccine

Contaminated with Simian Virus 40." *Journal of the National Cancer Institute* 95, no. 16 (2003): 1249.

DO VACCINES CAUSE DIABETES?

In 1990, the first *Haemophilus influenzae* type b (Hib) vaccine was licensed and recommended for all children in the United States (see the section titled "*Haemophilus influenzae* type b"). The vaccine was designed to prevent the twenty-five thousand cases of meningitis, pneumonia, and bloodstream infection that occurred in the United States every year. And it has. But when the vaccine was first licensed, it fell under a cloud of concern when a doctor named J. Bart Classen, speaking on the national television program *World News Tonight with Peter Jennings*, claimed that it caused diabetes.

Classen had compared children in Finland who had received the Hib vaccine at three, four, six, and fourteen months of age with those who had received it only at fourteen months of age. He reported finding that children who had received four doses were more likely to have diabetes than those who had received only one dose. Classen reasoned that the Hib vaccine was the cause. Other researchers tried to duplicate Classen's findings but couldn't. For example, one group of investigators followed thousands of children who had received the Hib vaccine for ten years and found no difference in the incidence of diabetes compared with thousands of children who hadn't received the vaccine.

Another group of investigators compared 250 people with diabetes with more than seven hundred without the disease to see whether those with diabetes were more likely to have received the pertussis, MMR, Hib, hepatitis B, or varicella vaccines. They weren't.

The inability of researchers to reproduce Classen's findings caused them to take a closer look at his study. They found that his analytical methods were incorrect. Hib-vaccinated infants, whether vaccinated with one or four doses, were no more likely than unvaccinated children to develop diabetes.

Therefore, the best available evidence does not support the notion that vaccines cause diabetes.

References

Black, Steven B., Edwin Lewis, Henry Shinefield, et al. "Lack of Association Between Receipt of Conjugate *Haemophilus Influenzae* Type B Vaccine (HbOC) in Infancy and Risk of Type 1 (Juvenile Onset) Diabetes: Long Term Follow-Up of the HbOC Efficacy Trial Cohort." *Pediatric Infectious Diseases Journal* 21, no. 6 (2002): 568–69.

DeStefano, Frank, John P. Mullooly, Catherine A. Okoro, et al. "Childhood Vaccinations, Vaccination Timing, and Risk of Type 1 Diabetes Mellitus." *Pediatrics* 108, no. 6 (2001): e112.

Institute for Vaccine Safety Diabetes Workshop Panel. "Childhood Immunizations and Type 1 Diabetes: Summary of an Institute for Vaccine Safety Workshop." *Pediatric Infectious Diseases Journal* 18, no. 3 (1999): 217–22.

DO VACCINES CAUSE MAD COW DISEASE?

Mad cow disease was a problem in the United Kingdom in the 1990s. Caused by unique infectious agents called proteinaceous infectious particles, or prions, it could spread to humans. The human form of mad cow disease, called variant Creutzfeldt-Jakob disease (vCJD), is a rapidly progressive, debilitating form of dementia. During the mad cow scare, some people became concerned that vaccines, which may contain trace amounts of animal products used in the manufacturing process, could cause vCJD.

Vaccines are grown in laboratory cells that require many factors for maintenance, some of which are obtained from animals. An excellent source of these growth factors is serum from the fetuses of cows (fetal bovine serum). Because of concerns about vCJD, the FDA prohibited the use of bovine-derived materials obtained from countries known to have a problem with mad cow disease. This raised the question of whether children inoculated with vaccines prior to the ban were at risk for vCJD. Newspapers reported this possibility in the late 1990s. However, several features of mad cow disease should reassure parents that vaccines never caused vCJD.

First, the prions that cause mad cow disease are detected in the brain, spinal cord, and retinas of cows, not in blood, serum, or other organs. Therefore, trace quantities of fetal bovine serum that might be present in liquids that support the growth of cells used to make vaccines don't contain prions. Indeed, no cases of vCJD have been caused by exposure to blood or blood products, and a history of blood transfusion does not increase a person's risk for vCJD.

Second, even in England, products used in vaccines that were derived from cows didn't cause vCJD. Studies clearly showed that children in England who had received vaccines were no more likely to develop vCJD than those who hadn't.

Third, prion transmission occurs by eating the brains of infected animals or, in experimental studies, directly inoculating preparations of brains from infected animals into the brains of healthy animals. Prion transmission has never been documented after inoculation into muscle or under the skin (routes used for vaccination).

Taken together, the chance that currently licensed vaccines cause vCJD is zero.

References

Brown, Paul. "Can Creutzfeldt-Jakob Disease Be Transmitted by Transfusion?" *Current Opinions in Hematology* 2, no. 6 (1995): 472–77.

Marwick, Charles. "FDA Calls Bovine-Based Vaccines Currently Safe." *Journal of the American Medical Association* 284, no. 10 (2000): 1231–32.

Minor, P. D., R. G. Will, and D. Salisbury. "Vaccines and Variant CJD." *Vaccine* 19, nos. 4–5 (2001): 409–10.

DO VACCINES CAUSE MULTIPLE SCLEROSIS?

Multiple sclerosis is a chronic disease of the brain caused when the immune system reacts against the lining of nerves.

Nerves are like electrical wires surrounded by thin rubber tubing. The sheath covering nerves is made of myelin, and the main component of myelin is myelin basic protein. People develop multiple sclerosis when cells of the immune system called T cells react to the myelin basic protein and destroy it. Although the root cause (or causes) of multiple sclerosis remains unclear, we know that it is an autoimmune disease involving an abnormal response to myelin.

In the mid-1980s, some people became concerned that the hepatitis B vaccine could cause an immune response against myelin that would result in multiple sclerosis. This fear became so widespread that the French government temporarily suspended its school-based hepatitis B vaccination program.

However, the idea that the hepatitis B vaccine caused multiple sclerosis was flawed for several reasons. First, there is only one protein in the hepatitis B vaccine (called the hepatitis B surface protein), and it doesn't mimic myelin basic protein, so an immune response to the vaccine shouldn't cause an immune response to myelin. Second, natural infection with hepatitis B virus is associated with the production of large quantities of hepatitis B surface protein—about ten thousand times more than contained in the vaccine—but is not associated with an increased risk of multiple sclerosis.

Further evidence that vaccines don't cause multiple sclerosis can be found in two large studies, both reported in the *New England Journal of Medicine*. The first involved hundreds of thousands of nurses observed for more than a decade. Nurses who developed multiple sclerosis were no more likely to have received the hepatitis B vaccine than those who didn't develop the disease. The second study, involving hundreds of people with multiple sclerosis in Europe, was conducted to determine whether the hepatitis B, influenza, or tetanus vaccines caused symptoms to worsen. They didn't.

Vaccines do not cause multiple sclerosis or worsen its symptoms.

References

Ascherio, Alberto, Shumin M. Zhang, Miguel A. Hernán, et al. "Hepatitis B Vaccination and the Risk of Multiple Sclerosis." *New England Journal of Medicine* 344, no. 5 (2001): 327–32.

Confavreux, Christian, Samy Suissa, Patricia Saddier, et al. "Vaccinations and the Risk of Relapse in Multiple Sclerosis." *New England Journal of Medicine* 344, no. 5 (2001): 319–26.

DO VACCINES CAUSE SUDDEN INFANT DEATH SYNDROME?

Every year in the United States, babies die of sudden infant death syndrome (SIDS), a disorder that is poorly understood and which primarily affects infants between two and four months of age. In the 1980s, some parents believed that the older version of the pertussis vaccine (called the "whole-cell" pertussis vaccine) was the cause. However, several studies compared the incidence of SIDS in babies who either had or hadn't received pertussis vaccine and found that babies who died from SIDS were not more likely to have received it.

In the early 1990s, the hypothesis shifted when a new vaccine—the hepatitis B vaccine—was recommended for babies. Around the time of the recommendation, the ABC news program *20/20* aired a story claiming that the vaccine caused SIDS. The reporter told the story of a one-month-old girl who had died of SIDS sixteen hours after receiving her second dose of the hepatitis B vaccine. At the time the story aired, about five thousand children died of SIDS annually. Within ten years of the introduction of the hepatitis B vaccine, about 90 percent of infants were immunized, and the incidence of SIDS decreased to about 1,600 cases a year. In other words, as the number of babies immunized against hepatitis B increased dramatically, the number of babies dying from SIDS decreased dramatically. However, despite this correlation, the cause of the decrease in the incidence of SIDS wasn't related to the increase in hepatitis B vaccination at all. Rather, it was discovered that infants who died of SIDS were more likely to have slept face down. In response, the American Academy of Pediatrics introduced the "Back to Sleep" program, which dramatically reduced the number of SIDS deaths.

Neither the pertussis vaccine nor the hepatitis B vaccine causes SIDS.

Reference

Griffin, Marie R., Wayne A. Ray, John R. Livengood, et al. "Risk of Sudden Infant Death Syndrome After Immunization with the Diphtheria-Tetanus-Pertussis Vaccine." *New England Journal of Medicine* 319, no. 10 (1988): 618–23.

DO VACCINES AFFECT FERTILITY?

Vaccines would not be expected to affect fertility for two reasons. First, if a vaccine-preventable disease does not affect fertility, the vaccine, which is a weakened or partial version of the pathogen, would not be likely to affect fertility either. Second, vaccines are typically processed by immune system cells near the site of administration. Despite these facts, fertility concerns related to a couple of vaccines have persisted.

HPV Vaccine

Although human papillomavirus (HPV) can affect a person's ability to reproduce (for example, if they develop cervical cancer), HPV infection does not lead directly to infertility. Additionally, the HPV vaccine contains only the surface protein from the HPV virus. So, the HPV vaccine would not be expected to cause fertility issues. However, the HPV vaccine has been suggested as a cause of primary ovarian failure, a condition in which the ovaries stop working earlier than usual, leading to early menopause. Because of these concerns, scientists evaluated whether receiving the HPV vaccine was associated with primary ovarian failure. These studies, which evaluated hundreds of thousands of HPV vaccine recipients demonstrated no link between receipt of the vaccine and primary ovarian failure.

COVID-19 mRNA Vaccines

The fear of COVID-19 vaccines causing infertility was spawned by Michael Yeadon, a retired researcher who had worked for Pfizer, and Wolfgang Wodarg, a physician, following the release of COVID-19 mRNA vaccines in 2021. Yeadon and Wodarg argued that the SARS-CoV-2 spike protein, which is made in the body following vaccination, was virtually identical to a protein called syncytin-1, which resides on the surface of placental cells. They believed that women making an immune response to the viral spike protein in an mRNA COVID-19 vaccine might also inadvertently make an immune response to their own placenta, causing infertility. As it turned out, the SARS-CoV-2 spike protein and syncytin-1 are immunologically distinct, so an immune response to one protein isn't necessarily an immune response to another.

Given that more than two hundred million people in the United States have been infected with SARS-CoV-2 and that all of them have made an immune response to the spike protein, if Yeadon and Wodarg were right, the birth rate during the COVID-19 pandemic should have plummeted. But it didn't. It remained the same. Other studies comparing women who had or hadn't received the COVID-19 mRNA vaccines also showed no difference in pregnancy outcomes.

References

Arana, Jorge E., Theresa Harrington, Maria Cano, et al. "Post-Licensure Safety Monitoring of Quadrivalent Human Papillomavirus Vaccine in the Vaccine Adverse Event Reporting System (VAERS), 2009–2015." *Vaccine* 36, no. 13 (2018) 1781–88.

Naleway, Allison L., Kathleen F. Mittendorf, Stephanie A. Irving, et al. "Primary Ovarian Insufficiency and Adolescent Vaccination." *Pediatrics* 142, no. 3 (2018): e20180943.

Shimabakuro, Tom T., Shin Y. Kim, Tanya R. Myers, et al. "Preliminary Findings of mRNA Covid-19 Vaccine Safety in Pregnant Persons," *New England Journal of Medicine* 384, no. 24 (2021) 2273–82.

Zaçe, D., E. La Gatta, L. Petrella, and M. L. Di Pietro, "The Impact of COVID-19 Vaccines on Fertility: A Systematic Review and Meta-Analysis," *Vaccine* 40, no. 42 (2022) 6023–34.

DO VACCINES CAUSE ANTIBODY-DEPENDENT ENHANCEMENT?

Our bodies respond to viral vaccines and viral infections by making antibodies that prevent the virus from attaching to and entering cells. These types of antibodies are called virus-neutralizing antibodies. But not all antibodies neutralize the virus that they are specific for. Some bind to parts of the virus that don't prevent it from attaching to and entering cells. These types of antibodies are called virus-binding antibodies.

It's possible for certain virus-binding antibodies to attach to a virus and actually facilitate its entrance into cells. This phenomenon is called antibody-dependent enhancement (ADE). The only vaccine-preventable virus, and the only viral vaccine, for which this occurs is the dengue vaccine. As a result, recommendations regarding the use of the dengue vaccine are limited to very specific groups of individuals (see "Dengue" section in the "Vaccines for 7- to 18-year-olds" chapter). The phenomenon of ADE does not occur for any other vaccine.

DO mRNA VACCINES CHANGE OUR DNA?

Because the COVID-19 mRNA vaccines were the first "genetic" vaccines, some people worried that they could alter DNA, but that is biologically impossible. Two aspects of this phenomenon have caused concerns.

The contextual biology

Our cells all have DNA and messenger RNA (mRNA). DNA is our genetic code. It is protected in the nucleus of our cells. From DNA, mRNA is made (called transcription) and released from the nucleus into the cytoplasm of the cell. Once in the cytoplasm, mRNA is processed to produce proteins (called translation). Our cells translate mRNA into proteins all the time.

Introduction of mRNA from a vaccine

The mRNA vaccines take advantage of the regular processing of mRNA by our cells, so that instead of delivering proteins via a vaccine that our immune systems respond to, our cells make the protein that our immune systems respond to. Concerns about vaccine-introduced mRNA changing our DNA are unfounded for three reasons. First, mRNA vaccines don't have the nuclear access signal that would allow mRNA to enter the nucleus of a cell where DNA resides: you can't alter DNA if you can't get to it. Second, mRNA vaccines don't have the enzyme (called reverse transcriptase) that would allow for conversion of the mRNA into DNA: you can't alter DNA if you don't have DNA. Third, even if mRNA from the vaccine could be converted to DNA, the vaccine doesn't have the enzyme (called integrase) that would allow integration into DNA; you can't alter DNA if you can't insert new DNA into existing DNA. As such, mRNA in the vaccines cannot cause changes to our DNA.

Introduction of DNA fragments from a vaccine

To make the mRNA for the vaccine, the DNA for the protein of interest (in the case of COVID-19 vaccines, the spike protein) is put into cells that reproduce and as they reproduce, more spike protein DNA is made. This DNA is then isolated, purified, and used to make the mRNA that is delivered in the vaccine. Because DNA is part of the production process, a second concern related to whether mRNA vaccines could change our DNA emerged. Specifically, people wondered if leftover fragments of DNA from the production process could change our DNA. Like with the mRNA in the vaccine, the enzymes necessary for the DNA fragments to insert into our DNA are not present. Further, the quantity of the DNA fragments is very small (i.e., billionths of a gram). Therefore, the DNA fragments in mRNA vaccines cannot cause changes to our DNA.

ARE THERE "HOT LOTS" OF VACCINES?

Vaccines are produced in batches or lots that vary in size from thousands to tens of thousands of doses. Each lot is assigned a number, which is then printed on the label of each vial of vaccine.

Some people wonder whether lot-to-lot variation could lead to variation in the safety of a particular vaccine, causing some lots to be less safe than others (i.e., "hot lots".) However, the FDA requires that representative samples of every lot of a vaccine be tested for consistency. Vaccine manufacturers must demonstrate that the vials of every lot contain the same amount of vaccine, buffering agents, stabilizing agents, residual cellular DNA, and cellular proteins, as well as the same potency. Although there have been serious problems with some vaccines, those weren't caused by lot-to-lot variation.

For example, in 1955 Cutter Laboratories produced a version of Jonas Salk's inactivated polio vaccine. Unfortunately, the polioviruses used weren't properly inactivated. Consequently, about 120,000 children were injected with live poliovirus: 164 were permanently paralyzed, and ten died. In response, vaccine regulatory systems were put in place at the National Institutes of Health (NIH) and later at the FDA to make sure that such a thing never happened again. And it hasn't. No vaccine has since been recalled because improper manufacturing caused a problem with safety. Although the RotaShield vaccine was withdrawn in 1999 after it was found, post-licensure, to cause intestinal blockage (see "What Systems Are in Place to Ensure Vaccines Are Safe?"), the problem had nothing to do with the way the vaccine was made.

References

Murphy, Trudy V., Paul M. Gargiullo, Mehran S. Massoudi, et al. "Intussusception Among Infants Given an Oral Rotavirus Vaccine." *New England Journal of Medicine* 344, no. 8 (2001): 564–72.

Offit, Paul A. *The Cutter Incident: How America's First Polio Vaccine Led to the Growing Vaccine Crisis.* New Haven, CT: Yale University Press, 2005.

IS THE VACCINE ADVERSE EVENT REPORTING SYSTEM EFFECTIVE?

As mentioned, suspected side effects of vaccines should be reported to the Vaccine Adverse Event Reporting System (VAERS), which is codirected by the FDA and the CDC. VAERS is an important vaccine safety monitoring system; however, its data are sometimes cited erroneously as evidence that vaccines are not safe. VAERS was created by the National Childhood Vaccine Injury Act passed by Congress in 1986. Probably the best example of how VAERS works is the short-lived rotavirus vaccine that was given to U.S. children between 1998 and 1999 (see "What Systems Are in Place to Ensure Vaccines Are Safe?"). After the vaccine, which was called RotaShield, had been on the market for about ten months and given to about a million children, VAERS received 15 reports of a rare intestinal blockage (called intussusception) within a week following receipt of the vaccine. This raised a red flag, but it didn't prove anything. Because one in 2,000 infants developed intussusception every year even before the RotaShield vaccine was licensed, the question was whether the vaccine caused intussusception or these cases were merely coincidental. The only way to find out was to perform a large study examining thousands of children who did or didn't receive the vaccine. When that was done, it became clear that children who had received RotaShield were more likely to develop intussusception than those who hadn't, so the vaccine was removed from the market.

The same series of events occurred following the release of COVID-19 mRNA vaccines at the end of 2020. VAERS reports of myocarditis (inflammation of the heart muscle) following receipt of COVID-19 vaccine starting accumulating. In response, studies were performed through the Vaccine Safety DataLink (VSD; see "What Systems Are in Place to Ensure that Vaccines Are Safe?"). The VSD studies, which included a control group unlike VAERS reports, showed that those who received the

COVID-19 mRNA vaccines were at greater risk of myocarditis than those who hadn't received the vaccine.

Because events reported to VAERS represent a temporal association between a vaccine and a problem and because reporting is voluntary and can be done by anyone, reports to this system cannot possibly determine whether a vaccine *caused* a problem.

For example, in 1999, VAERS began receiving many reports, primarily from personal injury lawyers, that thimerosal in vaccines caused autism (see "Do Vaccines Cause Autism?"). Subsequent studies showed that children who had received vaccines containing thimerosal weren't at greater risk for autism than those who received the same vaccines without thimerosal. As with the case of RotaShield, submissions to VAERS had sounded an alarm. But unlike with Rotashield, this time it was a false alarm. The thimerosal story points out the critical flaw of VAERS: whereas reports to VAERS can raise the possibility of a problem, they cannot determine whether a vaccine *caused* a problem. That's because VAERS never receives reports from two important groups: people with the problem who didn't receive the vaccine and people who received the vaccine but didn't develop the problem. Data from both groups are necessary to determine whether a vaccine causes a problem.

Another example of how VAERS can be misleading involves the HPV vaccine (see "Human Papillomavirus" section). Following widespread distribution of the vaccine after its release in 2006, VAERS received several reports claiming that it might have caused blood clots, strokes, and heart attacks. One group of people, however, doesn't report to VAERS: women who used birth control pills who had not received the vaccine. Because the vaccine is given to young women, because some young women take birth control pills, and because birth control pills can cause blood clots and consequent strokes and heart attacks, this was an important group to hear from. Later, investigators found that birth control pills, not the HPV vaccine, had caused the reported problems.

Despite their limitations, VAERS reports are occasionally presented to the public as evidence that vaccines cause harm. Stories in the media and social media posts often present VAERS reports as fact, which can be quite misleading. Although VAERS is a good first-alarm system, it alone cannot determine whether a vaccine has caused a problem. Other systems, like the VSD, are in place to do that.

References

Goodman, Michael J., and James Nordin. "Vaccine Adverse Event Reporting System Reporting Source: A Possible Source of Bias in Longitudinal Studies." *Pediatrics* 117, no. 2 (2006): 387–90.

Yih, W. Katherine, Matthew F. Daley, Jonathan Duffy, et al. "A Broad Assessment of COVID-19 Vaccine Safety Using Tree-Based Data-Mining in the Vaccine Safety Datalink," *Vaccine* 41, no. 3 (2023) 826–35.

ARE PACKAGE INSERTS USEFUL?

Package inserts contain important information about vaccines: for example, a list of ingredients, details of the studies performed to determine whether a vaccine is safe and effective, dosage information, special considerations for various groups, contraindications (i.e., who shouldn't get the vaccine), precautions (i.e., who might be at risk from the vaccine), and possible adverse reactions.

Unfortunately, one aspect of package inserts can be misleading. Studies to determine whether a vaccine is safe and effective typically include two groups: those who have received the vaccine and those who haven't. This is done so that researchers can determine whether the vaccine causes a problem. If more people who received the vaccine experience a particular side effect than those who didn't get the vaccine, the vaccine probably caused the problem. Conversely, if about the same number of people in each group experience a side effect, then the vaccine probably didn't cause the problem. Unfortunately, package inserts often state that a vaccine might cause a particular side effect even when it occurred with the same frequency in both vaccinated and unvaccinated study participants. This is probably because package inserts are written by pharmaceutical company lawyers who want to make sure that they haven't failed to warn people about possible side effects. For this reason, inserts are more like legal documents than medical ones and can be misleading to people trying to determine whether a vaccine may cause certain side effects.

HOW DO I SORT OUT THE GOOD INFORMATION ABOUT VACCINES FROM THE BAD?

People are often confronted with information on television, on the internet, in magazines and newspapers, on social media, and in books that conflicts with that provided by health care professionals. What to do? The best way to understand vaccines, how they work, and whether they are effective and safe is to read the scientific studies. For example, several hundred papers have been published in medical journals describing the chickenpox vaccine. Indeed, the standard vaccine textbook contains references to more than twenty thousand studies. To understand these studies, individuals would need a background in microbiology, immunology, epidemiology, and statistics. This knowledge would enable them to separate good scientific studies from poor ones. But few people—and frankly, few doctors—have this kind of expertise. So, doctors rely on the expert guidance of specialists with experience and training in these disciplines.

Such groups of experts are composed of scientists, clinicians, and other caregivers who are as passionately devoted to our health as they are to their own family's health. Examples include the following:

• The American Academy of Family Physicians: https://www.aafp.org
• The American Academy of Pediatrics: https://www.aap.org
• The American College of Obstetricians and Gynecologists: https://www.acog.org

- The Centers for Disease Control and Prevention: https://www.cdc.gov
- Immunize.org: https://www.immunize.org
- The Institute for Vaccine Safety at the Johns Hopkins Bloomberg School of Public Health: https://www.vaccinesafety.edu
- Vaccinate Your Family: https://www.vaccinateyourfamily.org
- The Vaccine Education Center at Children's Hospital of Philadelphia: https://www.chop.edu/centers-programs/vaccine-education-center
- Voices for Vaccines: https://www.voicesforvaccines.org

These groups provide excellent information to parents and health care professionals through their websites, print materials, videos, social media channels, and other programming. Their task is to determine whether scientific studies are performed carefully, published in reputable journals, and, most importantly, reproducible. Information that fails to meet these standards is unreliable.

References

Centers for Disease Control and Prevention. "Finding Credible Vaccine Information." Last reviewed September 15, 2021. https://www.cdc.gov/vaccines/vac-gen/evalwebs.htm.

Children's Hospital of Philadelphia. "Vaccine Science: Evaluating Scientific Information and Studies." Last reviewed May 20, 2020. https://www.chop.edu/centers-programs/vaccine-education-center/vaccine-science/evaluating-scientific-information-and-studies.

HOW CAN I TALK TO RELATIVES OR FRIENDS WITH DIFFERENT IDEAS ABOUT VACCINES?

When it comes to vaccines, we ask a lot from parents in the United States. During the first few years of life, children can receive as many as twenty-seven inoculations to prevent diseases that most people don't see using biological fluids that most people don't understand. It's not hard to understand why some parents could fear all these shots. So, the most important thing when talking to friends or family members is to be understanding. It is perfectly reasonable to be skeptical of anything that we put into our bodies, especially vaccines given to healthy young children.

When people have fears about vaccines, it's usually because they're worried about vaccine safety. For example, after the scare about the MMR vaccine potentially causing autism in the late 1990s (see "Do Vaccines Cause Autism?"), thousands of parents refused to have their children receive the MMR vaccine, resulting in hundreds of hospitalizations and several deaths from measles. Despite the millions of dollars that went into research that confirmed there was no evidence that the MMR vaccine caused autism, some people remained skeptical. And some had crossed the line from skepticism to cynicism, believing in a vast international conspiracy of researchers hiding the truth. Likely nothing will reassure those who have fallen into this group.

However, people hearing the concerns of others should evaluate the arguments for themselves and consider whether the individual sharing it is someone who is unwilling to be convinced by high-quality evidence or if the individual may be motivated by something other than a true concern for people's health.

The Vaccine Education Center at Children's Hospital of Philadelphia provides helpful resources to address people's vaccine concerns, including the following:

- "Evaluating Information": https://media.chop.edu/data/files/pdfs /vaccine-education-center-evaluating-info-qa.pdf
- "Families and Vaccines: When Opinions Differ": https://media.chop .edu/data/files/pdfs/families-vaccines.pdf
- "Logical Fallacies and Vaccines": https://media.chop.edu/data/files /pdfs/vaccine-education-center-logical-fallacies.pdf

INGREDIENTS

DO VACCINES CONTAIN ALLERGENS?

The Centers for Disease Control and Prevention (CDC) estimates that every year several substances in vaccines cause about two hundred people in the United States to experience severe allergic reactions.

Egg Proteins

About one of two hundred people in the United States is allergic to eggs. Most are only mildly allergic, but some are severely allergic. Symptoms of a severe allergic reaction include hives, difficulty breathing, and low blood pressure. Because some influenza vaccines are made in eggs, egg proteins are present in some of the final products, usually in an amount measured in micrograms (i.e., millionths of a gram) per dose. Although current influenza vaccines contain trace quantities of egg proteins, these quantities are too small to cause an allergic reaction, even in people with severe egg allergies. Therefore, people with severe egg allergies can receive influenza vaccines safely.

The other vaccine grown in eggs is the yellow fever vaccine. Unfortunately, the quantity of egg proteins in this vaccine is large enough to cause a severe allergic reaction in people who are severely allergic to eggs. For this reason, people with severe egg allergies should avoid the yellow fever vaccine.

Some people think that if they're allergic to eggs, they can't get the measles-mumps-rubella (MMR) vaccine. But none of the viruses in the MMR vaccine are made in eggs; they're made in chick embryo cells, grown in culture in the laboratory. The quantity of residual egg proteins found in the MMR vaccine is measured in picograms (i.e., trillionths of a gram). Such a quantity is at least five hundred times less than that found in the yellow fever vaccine, so it doesn't cause a problem. Therefore, people allergic to eggs can safely receive the MMR vaccine.

DID YOU KNOW?

One raisin weighs about a gram, so a microgram is about one-millionth (0.000001) the weight of a raisin, and a picogram is about one-trillionth (0.000000000001) the weight of a raisin.

Antibiotics

Antibiotics are present in some vaccines to prevent bacterial contamination during the manufacturing process. Fortunately, the antibiotics most likely to cause allergic reactions, like penicillins, cephalosporins, and sulfa drugs, aren't contained in vaccines. Antibiotics used during vaccine manufacture include neomycin, streptomycin, polymyxin B, chlortetracycline, and amphotericin B. However, only neomycin is contained in vaccines in quantities large enough to be of potential concern. And severe allergic reactions to neomycin have not been found.

Yeast Proteins

Both the hepatitis B and human papillomavirus (HPV) vaccines contain yeast proteins. These vaccines are made by inserting the gene that makes one viral surface protein into a plasmid (a small circular piece of DNA) and putting the plasmid into baker's yeast. When the yeast cells grow, they also make the viral surface protein that eventually becomes the vaccine. The hepatitis B and HPV vaccines contain between 1 and 5 milligrams (thousandths of a gram) of yeast proteins.

Although some people are allergic to bread or bread products, it's not the yeast they're allergic to. No clear evidence exists that yeast proteins can induce the kind of immune responses necessary to cause severe allergic reactions. Therefore, the risk of experiencing a severe allergic reaction to baker's yeast is only theoretical.

Gelatin

In 1993, a seventeen-year-old girl in California developed a runny nose, hives, difficulty breathing, light-headedness, and low blood pressure within five minutes of receiving an MMR vaccine. When later describing the event, she said that it was "kind of like what happens when I eat Jell-O." Subsequent testing by an allergist found that the only substance in the vaccine to which the girl was allergic was gelatin, the main ingredient in Jell-O.

Gelatin, made by extracting collagen (the most abundant protein in the body) from the skin and hooves of pigs, is used in vaccines as a stabilizing agent, allowing small quantities of live viral vaccines to be evenly distributed throughout the vial.

The incidence of severe allergic reactions to gelatin is very low (about one case per two million doses), but it's still the most common identifiable cause of severe allergic reactions to vaccines. The gelatin in the MMR, chickenpox, and nasal spray influenza vaccines has been broken down with water molecules, so it is less likely to cause an allergic reaction. The gelatin found in the yellow fever vaccine and one rabies vaccine (Rabavert) is in a more natural form. Because of the low incidence of reactions and the low quantities present, it is hard to know whether the gelatin in vaccines can trigger a severe allergic reaction. However, some people have a history of allergies to gelatin-containing foods and are therefore more likely to experience an allergic rection to a vaccine containing gelatin. But even in this case, the gelatin in foods comes from cows, whereas that in vaccines comes from pigs, so people with a gelatin allergy should discuss the relative risks and benefits of gelatin-containing vaccines with their health care provider or an allergist.

References

GENERAL

Kelso, John M., James T. Li, Richard A. Nicklas, et al. "Adverse Reactions to Vaccines." *Annals of Allergy, Asthma, and Immunology* 103, no. 4, suppl. 2 (2009): S1–14.
Offit, Paul A., and R. K. Jew. "Addressing Parents' Concerns: Do Vaccines Contain Harmful Preservatives, Adjuvants, Additives, or Residuals?" *Pediatrics* 112, no. 6 (2003): 1394–97.

EGG PROTEINS

Bierman, C. Warren, Gail G. Shapiro, William E. Pierson, et al. "Safety of Influenza Vaccination in Allergic Children." *Journal of Infectious Diseases* 136 (1977): S652–55.
Fasano, Mary Beth, Robert A. Wood, Sara K. Cooke, and Hugh A. Sampson. "Egg Hypersensitivity and Adverse Reactions to Measles, Mumps, and Rubella Vaccine." *Journal of Pediatrics* 120, no. 6 (1992): 878–81.
Glezen, W. Paul. "Serious Morbidity and Mortality Associated with Influenza Epidemics." *Epidemiological Reviews* 4, no. 1 (1982): 25–44.
Glezen, W. Paul, Stephen B. Greenberg, Robert L. Atmar, et al. "Impact of Respiratory Virus Infection on Persons with Underlying Conditions." *Journal of the American Medical Association* 283, no. 4 (2000): 499–505.
Greenhawt, Matthew, Paul J. Turner, and John M. Kelso. "Administration of Influenza Vaccines to Egg Allergic Recipients: A Practice Parameter Update 2017," *Annals of Allergy, Asthma & Immunology* 120, no. 1 (2018): 49–52.
James, John M., A. Wesley Burks, Paula K. Roberson, and Hugh A. Sampson. "Safe Administration of the Measles Vaccine to

Children Allergic to Eggs." *New England Journal of Medicine* 332, no. 19 (1995): 1262–66.

James, John M., Robert S. Zeiger, Mitchell R. Lester, et al. "Safe Administration of Influenza Vaccine to Patients with Egg Allergy." *Journal of Pediatrics* 133, no. 5 (1998): 624–28.

Murphy, Kevin R., and Robert C. Strunk. "Safe Administration of Influenza Vaccine in Asthmatic Children Hypersensitive to Egg Proteins." *Journal of Pediatrics* 106, no. 6 (1985): 931–33.

Ratner, Bret, and Samuel Untracht. "Egg Allergy in Children: Incidence and Evaluation in Relation to Chick-Embryo-Propagated Vaccines." *American Journal of Diseases of Children* 83, no. 3 (1952): 309–16.

Smith, Derek, Priscilla Wong, Robert Gomez, and Kevin White. "Ovalbumin Content in the Yellow Fever Vaccine," *Journal of Allergy and Clinical Immunology Practice* 3, no. 5 (2015): 794–95.

Zieger, Robert S. "Current Issues with Influenza Vaccination in Egg Allergy." *Journal of Allergy and Clinical Immunology* 110, no. 6 (2002): 834–40.

ANTIBIOTICS

Anderson, John A., and N. Franklin Adkinson. "Allergic Reactions to Drugs and Biologic Agents." *Journal of the American Medical Association* 258, no. 20 (1987): 2891–99.

Goh, C. L. "Anaphylaxis from Topical Neomycin and Bacitracin." *Australasian Journal of Dermatology* 27, no. 3 (1986): 125–26.

Kwittken, Pamela L., Shea Rosen, and Sharon K. Sweinberg. "MMR Vaccine and Neomycin Allergy." *American Journal of Diseases of Children* 147, no. 2 (1993): 128–29.

Leyden, James J., and Albert M. Kligman. "Contact Dermatitis to Neomycin Sulfate." *Journal of the American Medical Association* 242, no. 12 (1979): 1276–78.

MacDonald, R. H., and M. Beck. "Neomycin: A Review with Particular Reference to Dermatological Usage." *Clinical Experimental Dermatology* 8, no. 3 (1983): 249–58.

Yunginger, John W. "Anaphylaxis." *Current Problems in Pediatrics* 22, no. 3 (1992): 130–46.

YEAST PROTEINS

Barbaud, A., P. Tréchot, S. Reichert-Pénétrat, et al. "Allergic Mechanisms and Urticaria/Angioedema After Hepatitis B Immunization." *British Journal of Dermatology* 139, no. 5 (1998): 925–26.

Brightman, C. A., G. K. Scadding, L. A. Dumbreck, et al. "Yeast-Derived Hepatitis B Vaccine and Yeast Sensitivity." *Lancet* 1, no. 8643 (1989): 903.

Hudson, Thomas J., Marianna Newkirk, Francine Gervais, and Joseph Shuster. "Adverse Reaction to the Recombinant Hepatitis B Vaccine." *Journal of Allergy and Clinical Immunology* 88, no. 5 (1991): 821–22.

Lear, J. T., and J. S. English. "Anaphylaxis After Hepatitis B Immunization." *Lancet* 345, no. 8959 (1995): 1249.

Wiederman, G., O. Scheiner, F. Ambrosch, et al. "Lack of Induction of IgE and IgG Antibodies to Yeast in Humans Immunized with Recombinant Hepatitis B Vaccines." *International Archives of Allergy and Applied Immunology* 85, no. 1 (1988): 130–32.

GELATIN

Kelso, John M., R. T. Jones, and J. W. Yunginger. "Anaphylaxis to Measles, Mumps, and Rubella Vaccine Mediated by IgE to Gelatin." *Journal of Allergy and Clinical Immunology* 91, no. 4 (1993): 867–72.

Sakaguchi, Masahiro, Hideo Ogura, and Sakae Inouye. "IgE Antibody to Gelatin in Children with Immediate-Type Reactions to Measles and Mumps Vaccines." *Journal of Allergy and Clinical Immunology* 96, no. 4 (1995): 563–65.

DO VACCINES CONTAIN HARMFUL PRESERVATIVES LIKE MERCURY?

The preservative in vaccines that has probably caused the most concern among parents is thimerosal. That's because thimerosal contains mercury, and large quantities of mercury can be toxic to the nervous system. The use of thimerosal in vaccines isn't new; mercury-containing preservatives have been in vaccines for decades.

Between 1900 and 1930, companies packaged vaccines almost exclusively in multidose vials, typically containing ten doses. This allowed the vaccines to be made much less expensively. Doctors kept the vials in refrigerators in their offices, often for months at a time. To give a vaccine, they would insert a needle through the rubber stopper, pull the liquid up into a syringe, and inject it. Unfortunately, by repeatedly inserting needles through the rubber stopper, doctors and nurses occasionally (and unintentionally) contaminated the vial with bacteria or fungi. In the early 1900s, many children developed local abscesses or serious bloodstream infections, including sepsis and death, caused by bacteria like *Staphylococcus* and *Streptococcus* that had contaminated the last few doses in the vial. By the 1940s, most multidose vials of vaccines contained preservatives like thimerosal to prevent contamination.

For decades, thimerosal was used in vaccines without a second thought. But as health officials added more vaccines to the routine schedule, children received more and more mercury. By the spring of 2001, the American Academy of Pediatrics and the U.S. Public Health Service decided to remove thimerosal from virtually all vaccines routinely recommended for children. While preservative levels of thimerosal are still contained in multidose preparations of the inactivated influenza vaccine, thimerosal hasn't been in vaccines routinely given to children since 2001. Unfortunately, the demand for the rapid removal of thimerosal caused some parents to wonder whether it had caused harm, specifically autism or subtle forms of mercury toxicity. Because mercury at high doses can be toxic to the nervous system, this concern was reasonable.

At the time of thimerosal's removal from vaccines, several facts about mercury were reassuring. Mercury is part of the earth's surface, released into the environment by burning coal, rock erosion, and volcanoes. After it's released, it settles onto the surface of lakes, rivers, and oceans, where it is converted to methylmercury by bacteria. Methylmercury is everywhere—in the fish we eat, the water we drink, and the infant formula and breast milk we feed our babies. There is no avoiding it. Because everyone drinks water, everyone has small amounts of methylmercury in their blood, urine, and hair. In fact, a typical breast-fed infant will ingest almost 400 micrograms (millionths of a gram) of methylmercury during the first six months of life. That's more than twice the amount of mercury than was ever contained in all childhood vaccines combined. And because the type of mercury in breast milk (methylmercury) is excreted from the body much more slowly than that contained in vaccines (ethylmercury), mercury ingested through breast milk is much more likely to accumulate in the body. This doesn't mean that breast milk or infant formula are dangerous. It means only that anyone who lives on the planet consumes small amounts of mercury all the time.

To address parents' concerns about whether thimerosal in vaccines caused harm, investigators in several countries compared children who had received thimerosal-containing vaccines with those who had received the same vaccines with smaller amounts of thimerosal or no thimerosal. They found no difference in the risk of autism among these groups. Further, children who had received thimerosal-containing vaccines didn't develop even subtle signs of mercury toxicity.

The use of a mercury-containing preservative in vaccines harkens back to a statement made by a seventeenth-century chemist named Paracelsus: "The dose makes the poison." In other words, although large quantities of a particular substance might be harmful, small quantities aren't. Indeed, we all have very small quantities of a variety of heavy metals in our bodies, including arsenic, cadmium, thallium, beryllium, and lead. All these substances can be harmful in large quantities, but the small quantities we encounter from typical exposure to these metals don't pose a risk.

References

Andrews, Nick, Elizabeth Miller, Andrew Grant, et al. "Thimerosal Exposure in Infants and Developmental Disorders: A Retrospective Cohort Study in the United Kingdom Does Not Support a Causal Association." *Pediatrics* 114, no. 3 (2004): 584–91.

Fombonne, Eric, Rita Zakarian, Andrew Bennett, et al. "Pervasive Developmental Disorders in Montreal, Quebec, Canada: Prevalence and Links with Immunization." *Pediatrics* 118, no. 1 (2006): e139–50.

Heron, Jon, and Jean Golding. "Thimerosal Exposure in Infants and Developmental Disorders: A Prospective Cohort Study in the United Kingdom Does Not Support a Causal Association." *Pediatrics* 114, no. 3 (2004): 577–83.

Hviid, Anders, Michael Stellfeld, Jan Wohlfahrt, and Mads Melbye. "Association Between Thimerosal-Containing Vaccine and Autism." *Journal of the American Medical Association* 290, no. 13 (2003): 1763–66.

Institute of Medicine. *Immunization Safety Review: Thimerosal-Containing Vaccines and Neurodevelopmental Disorders.* Washington, DC: National Academies Press, 2001.

Institute of Medicine. *Immunization Safety Review: Vaccines and Autism.* Washington, DC: National Academies Press, 2004.

Madsen, Kreesten M., Marlene B. Lauritsen, Carsten B. Pedersen, et al. "Thimerosal and the Occurrence of Autism: Negative Ecological Evidence from Danish Population-Based Data." *Pediatrics* 112, no. 3 (2003): 604–6.

Schechter, Robert, and Judith K. Grether. "Continuing Increases in Autism Reported to California's Development Services System." *Archives of General Psychiatry* 65, no. 1 (2008): 19–24.

Stehr-Green, Paul, Peet Tull, Michael Stellfeld, et al. "Autism and Thimerosal-Containing Vaccines: Lack of Consistent Evidence for an Association." *American Journal of Preventive Medicine* 25, no. 2 (2005): 101–6.

Thompson, William W., Cristofer Price, Barbara Goodson, et al. "Early Thimerosal Exposure and Neuropsychological Outcomes at 7 to 10 Years." *New England Journal of Medicine* 357, no. 13 (2007): 1281–92.

DO VACCINES CONTAIN HARMFUL ADJUVANTS LIKE ALUMINUM?

Adjuvants, which have been used in vaccines since the 1930s, were added to vaccines to enhance the immune response, allowing for lesser quantities and fewer doses of vaccine. (*Adjuvant* comes from the Latin *adjuvare*, meaning "to help.") The DTaP, hepatitis A, hepatitis B, Hib, RSV, pneumococcal, shingles, and one of the one of the COVID-19 vaccines (Novavax), all contain adjuvants.

Aluminum

Historically, vaccines contained only one type of adjuvant: aluminum salts. So, the safety of aluminum in vaccines has been assessed for more than eight decades. Some parents, however, are concerned that excess aluminum might cause harm. The facts are reassuring.

The amount of aluminum contained in vaccines is far less than that which babies typically face every day. That's because aluminum, the third most abundant element on Earth, is everywhere: in the air we breathe, the food we eat, and the water we drink. The most common source of aluminum is food. It's present naturally in teas, herbs, and spices. It's also added to leavening agents, anticaking agents, emulsifiers, and coloring agents. Large quantities of aluminum are found in pancake mixes, self-rising flours, baking powder, processed cheeses, and corn bread.

Because aluminum is everywhere, adults typically ingest between 5 and 10 milligrams (thousandths of a gram) of it every day. Babies are no different; all are exposed to aluminum in breast milk and infant formula. Those exclusively breast fed will ingest about 10 milligrams of aluminum by six months of age; those fed regular infant formula, 30 to 40 milligrams; and those fed soy formula, about 120 milligrams. These quantities are much greater than those contained in vaccines: babies who get all the recommended vaccines will receive about 4 milligrams of aluminum in the first six months of life.

Large quantities of aluminum—much greater than those contained in vaccines—can be harmful, causing brain dysfunction, weakening of the bones, and anemia. But harm from aluminum occurs in only two groups: severely premature infants who receive large quantities of aluminum in intravenous fluids and people on chronic dialysis for kidney failure who receive large quantities of aluminum in antacids. So, the only way babies can be harmed by aluminum is if their kidneys work poorly or not at all and if, at the same time, they are receiving large quantities of aluminum from intravenous fluids or medications like antacids. A typical antacid contains about 350 milligrams of aluminum per teaspoon.

Some people worry about the aluminum in vaccines because while only a small amount of aluminum that is ingested makes it into the bloodstream, all of the aluminum that is injected ends up in the bloodstream. However, when our body is processing chemicals, it does not distinguish where the chemical came from, so aluminum in the blood is processed the same regardless of whether it was eaten or injected. And even though the amount may be higher after vaccination, the body is capable of processing it, except in rare instances when, as previously described, the kidneys are not functioning properly and the quantities of aluminum are significant and introduced regularly over long periods of time (months or years).

Studies of aluminum in vaccines have also been reassuring. Because aluminum is unavoidable, everyone has it circulating in their bodies, even babies who have between 1 and 5 nanograms (billionths of a gram) per milliliter of blood. Researchers have studied whether vaccines containing aluminum increase the amount of aluminum in the blood. They don't. The quantity of aluminum in vaccines is so small that the amount in blood is unchanged after vaccination. Other studies have shown that the body eliminates aluminum quickly; in fact, about half of it is eliminated in just one day.

Monophosphoryl Lipid A and Saponin

Other adjuvants are also used in vaccines. The shingles vaccine and one of the RSV vaccines (AREXVY) contain a combination of adjuvants called monophosphoryl lipid A (MPLA) and saponin. Saponin is a soap. MPLA is a substance found on the surface of bacteria. When our body identifies something that resembles bacteria, our innate immune system springs into action. Both MPLA and saponin, when used as adjuvants, can cause low-grade fever and pain and redness at the injection site.

CpG

Another adjuvant, used in one of the hepatitis B vaccines (Heplisav-B), is called CpG, which stands for "cytosine and guanine linked by a phosphodiester." Cytosine and guanine, along with adenine and thymine, are building blocks of DNA. Bacterial DNA is composed of repeated units of cytosine and guanine, which do not occur in human DNA. Like MPLA, CpG stimulates the innate immune system, making for a powerful and safe adjuvant.

References

Institute for Vaccine Safety. "Excipients in Routinely Recommended Vaccines." Last updated August 31, 2023. https://www.vaccinesafety .edu/components-excipients/.

Keith, L. S., D. E. Jones, and C. Chou. "Aluminum Toxicokinetics Regarding Infant Diet and Vaccinations." *Vaccine* 20 (2002): S13–17.

Lal, Himal, Anthony L. Cunningham, Olivier Godeaux, et al., "Efficacy of an Adjuvanted Herpes Subunit Vaccine in Older Adults," *New England Journal of Medicine* 372, no. 22 (2015) 2087–96.

Offit, Paul A., and Rita K. Jew. "Addressing Parents' Concerns: Do Vaccines Contain Harmful Preservatives, Adjuvants, Additives, or Residuals?" *Pediatrics* 112, no. 6 (2003): 1394–1401.

Shirodkar, S., R. L. Hutchinson, D. L. Perry, et al. "Aluminum Compounds Used as Adjuvants in Vaccines." *Pharmacology Research* 7, no. 12 (1990): 1282–88.

Simmer, K., A. Fudge, J. Teubner, and S. L. James. "Aluminum Concentrations in Infant Milk Formulae." *Journal of Paediatric Child Health* 26, no. 1 (1990): 9–11.

Ushach, Irina, Ren Zhu, Elen Rosler, et al. "Targeting TLR9 Agonists to Secondary Lymphoid Organs Induces Potent Immune Responses Against HBV Infection," *Molecular Therapy: Nucleic Acids* 27 (2022) 1103–15.

Weintraub, R., G. Hams, M. Meerkin, and A. R. Rosenberg. "High Aluminum Content of Infant Milk Formulas." *Archives of Disease in Childhood* 61, no. 9 (1986): 914–16.

DO VACCINES CONTAIN HARMFUL CHEMICALS LIKE FORMALDEHYDE?

Vaccines are complicated to make. They're not like other pharmaceuticals for which the synthesis of small molecules can be performed relatively easily in a laboratory. Vaccines are biologicals, meaning they are made from organisms, so they are more complex to manufacture. Viruses can be grown only in cells; bacteria need nutrients to grow, and even for vaccines made using recombinant DNA technology (see "How Are Vaccines Made?")—like the hepatitis B and HPV vaccines—cells are still required to make the viral proteins used in the vaccine. Vaccines must also be sterile, so the process often involves the use of antibiotics (see "Do Vaccines Contain Products to Which People Could Be Allergic?").

Even after vaccines are made, they might require stabilizing agents, like gelatin, to ensure that the vaccine virus is equally distributed throughout the vial and doesn't stick to the sides. And vaccines require buffering agents to keep them stable across a wide range of temperatures.

Because of these requirements, vaccines may contain small quantities of fetal bovine serum (see "Do Vaccines Cause Mad

Cow Disease?"), monosodium glutamate, polysorbate, phenoxy-ethanol, ethylenediaminetetraacetic acid (EDTA), polyethylene glycol, sodium borate, octoxynol, and sodium deoxycholate. However, these chemicals are present only in very small amounts, and similar or greater quantities of them are found in foods, beverages, toothpastes, and over-the-counter medicines. But one particular chemical in vaccines has drawn much attention: formaldehyde.

Formaldehyde is used to inactivate viruses (like polio and hepatitis A) and bacterial toxins (like diphtheria and tetanus toxins); therefore, small quantities of formaldehyde are found in the final products. In addition to the chemical's use by morticians, conjuring up images of death, concerns have centered on the fact that large quantities of formaldehyde can damage cellular DNA, causing cancerous changes in cells grown in laboratory flasks.

Studies evaluating the potential for formaldehyde to cause cancer in people have had mixed results; however, the studies tended to focus on individuals exposed to large amounts of formaldehyde for long periods of time (years), typically resulting from occupational exposures, such as in the case of embalmers. In such individuals, the associated types of cancers include those of the nasopharynx and leukemia, specifically myeloid leukemia. Importantly, even in people with regular exposure over many years, the link between formaldehyde and cancer has not been found consistently. Although these studies led to formaldehyde being categorized as a carcinogen (a cancer-causing agent), the quantities used in vaccines are nowhere near those to which the study populations were exposed. Further, animals exposed to quantities of formaldehyde exponentially greater than those contained in vaccines don't develop malignancies. Indeed, quantities of formaldehyde at least six hundred times greater than those contained in vaccines have been given safely to animals.

The quantity of formaldehyde in individual vaccines does not exceed one-tenth of a milligram (thousandths of a gram). This amount is safe for several reasons. First, formaldehyde is one of the intermediary products of human metabolism and a necessary component in the synthesis of thymidine, purines, and amino acids, which are necessary for the formation of DNA and proteins. Therefore, everyone has detectable quantities of formaldehyde in their bloodstream, about 2.5 micrograms (millionths of a gram) of formaldehyde per milliliter (one-fifth of a teaspoon) of blood. Assuming an average two-month-old weighs 5 kilograms (about eleven pounds) and has a blood volume of 85 milliliters per kilogram, the total amount of formaldehyde found naturally in their circulation would be about 1 milligram—a value at least ten times that contained in any individual vaccine. In other words, there is far more formaldehyde circulating naturally in our bodies than contained in vaccines.

References

Goldmacher, Victor S., and William G. Thilly. "Formaldehyde Is Mutagenic for Cultured Human Cells." *Mutation Research* 116, nos. 3–4 (1983): 417–22.

Heck, Henry D., Mercedes Casanova-Schmitz, Parker B. Dodd, et al. "Formaldehyde (CH_2O) Concentrations in the Blood of Humans and Fischer-344 Rats Exposed to CH_2O Under Controlled Conditions." *American Industrial Hygiene Association Journal* 46, no. 1 (1985): 1–3.

Huennekens, F. M., and M. J. Osborne. "Folic Acid Coenzymes and One-Carbon Metabolism." *Advances in Enzymology* 21 (1959): 369–446.

Natarajan, A. T., F. Darroudi, C. J. M. Bussman, and A. C. van Kesteren-van Leeuwen. "Evaluation of the Mutagenicity of Formaldehyde in Mammalian Cytogenetic Assays In Vivo and In Vitro." *Mutation Research* 122, nos. 3–4 (1983): 355–60.

Ragan, Daniel L., and Craig J. Boreiko. "Initiation of $C3H/10T1/2$ Cell Transformation by Formaldehyde." *Cancer Letters* 13, no. 4 (1981): 325–31.

Tepper, L. B. "Epidemiology of Chronic Occupational Exposure to Formaldehyde: Report of the Ad Hoc Panel on Health Aspects of Formaldehyde." *Toxicology and Industrial Health* 4, no. 1 (1988): 77–90.

Til, H. P., R. A. Woutersen, V. J. Feron, et al. "Two-Year Drinking-Water Study of Formaldehyde in Rats." *Food and Chemical Toxicology* 27, no. 2 (1989): 77–87.

DO VACCINES CONTAIN ETHER OR ANTIFREEZE?

The concern that vaccines contain ether or antifreeze has been propagated on the internet as well as by antivaccine celebrities on national television shows and social media.

Ether is the common name given to the chemical diethyl ether, an anesthetic no longer used in hospitals in large part because it is highly flammable. Vaccines don't contain diethyl ether. It's hard to know why this myth started, but it might be because manufacturers use small amounts of a mild detergent to break open the cells used to grow vaccine viruses. This mild detergent has the chemical name polyethylene glycol pisooctylphenyl ether. Ethers are organic compounds that link carbohydrates via a central oxygen atom. They are commonly found in nature, so we are exposed to these harmless chemicals every day.

Antifreeze is used to prevent water from freezing, primarily in car engines. Quaker State AntiFreeze and Coolant is typical of most products, containing ethylene glycol and diethylene glycol. Sometimes antifreeze products contain methanol, also known as wood alcohol. Vaccines don't contain any of these chemicals. Again, it's hard to figure out where this notion came from, but it may have to do with the presence of trace amounts of the harmless chemical polyethylene glycol, which is not antifreeze and is often found in other products, such as over-the-counter medicines and toothpastes.

ARE VACCINES MADE USING ABORTED FETAL CELLS?

Viruses and bacteria are different. Whereas bacteria can grow on the surface of the skin, nose, or throat, viruses can grow only inside cells. So, when making viral vaccines, cells are a required part of the process. One of the advantages of using human fetal cells is that they are essentially immortal; they can reproduce many, many times before dying. This is in direct contrast with cells obtained from organs that are fully developed; such cells reproduce about fifty times before they can no longer be used. Because fetal cells are longer-lived, they can be used to make viral vaccines for centuries.

Other aspects of human fetal cells also make them attractive for vaccine use. First, human cells are much more likely to support the growth of human viruses than are animal cells. Second, because the fetus is in a sterile environment, human fetal cells are sterile, meaning they're not contaminated with other viruses. This typically isn't the case with cells obtained from live animals or humans after birth.

In the early 1960s, cells used to make vaccines were obtained from two elective abortions—one performed in Sweden, the other in England. The human fetal cells obtained from Sweden were sent to the Wistar Institute in Philadelphia, where Dr. Stanley Plotkin was working on a rubella vaccine and Dr. Tad Wiktor was working on a rabies vaccine. These cells were called Wistar Institute-38 or WI-38 cells. The cells obtained in England were studied at the United Kingdom's Medical Research Council; they're called MRC-5 cells. These two sources of human fetal cells have been used to make vaccines against rubella, rabies, chickenpox, and hepatitis A.

More recently, the adenovirus-based COVID-19 vaccines (like the one made by Janssen/Johnson & Johnson) were also made using fetal cells. The adenovirus strain used in vaccine production cannot replicate in people, so to produce the vaccine, the adenovirus containing the gene of interest (in this case the SARS-CoV-2 spike protein) must be grown in a cell line that includes a gene that will enable it to reproduce. A retinal cell line, called PER.C6, was isolated in the mid-1980s and adapted to include the necessary gene for this application. (The Janssen/Johnson & Johnson vaccine is no longer used in the United

States because of some rare but severe side effects and the availability of other COVID-19 vaccines.)

To some, using human fetal cells to make vaccines is abhorrent, an act against God. In July 2005, in response to pressures from a pro-life group in the United States, the Vatican's Pontifical Academy for Life ruled on whether using vaccines derived from human fetal cells was wrong. The ruling was made by Cardinal Joseph Ratzinger, then the head of the Catholic Church's Congregation for the Doctrine of the Faith. Ratzinger was a well-known theologian and prolific author. He later became Pope Benedict XVI, the 265th pope (until he retired in February 2013). Ratzinger reasoned that those involved in the original abortion had "formally cooperated with evil." But he decided that the doctors and nurses who give vaccines made from human fetal cells are engaged in only a "very, very remote" form of cooperation with evil, so remote that "it does not indicate any [negative] moral value" when compared with the greater good of preventing life-threatening infections.

The National Catholic Bioethics Center agreed with the Vatican's decision: "Clearly the use of a vaccine in the present does not cause the one who is immunized to share in the immoral intention or action of those who carried out the abortion in the past. . . . Human history is filled with injustice. Acts of wrongdoing in the past regularly redound to the benefit of descendants who had no hand in the original crimes. It would be a high standard indeed if we were to require all benefits that we receive in the present to be completely free of every immorality in the past."

References

Furton, Edward J. "Vaccines Originating in Abortion." *Ethics and Medics* 24, no. 3 (1999): 3–4.

Glatz, C. "Vatican Says Refusing Vaccines Must Be Weighed Against Health Threats." Catholic News Service. http://www.catholicnews.com/data/stories/cns/0504240.htm.

Offit, P. A. *Vaccinated: One Man's Quest to Defeat the World's Deadliest Diseases.* New York: Smithsonian Books, 2007.

Pontifical Academy for Life, Congregation for the Doctrine of the Faith. "Moral Reflection on Vaccines Prepared from Cells Derived from Aborted Human Foetuses." Protection of Conscience Project. http://www.consciencelaws.org/Conscience-Policies-Papers/PPPCatholico3.html.

Pontificia Academia Pro Vita. "Vatican Statement on Vaccines Derived from Aborted Human Fetuses." Immunize.org. http://www.immunize.org/concerns/vaticandocument.htm.

DO VACCINES CONTAIN ANIMAL PRODUCTS?

Some viral vaccines are made in animal cells (for example, monkey kidney cells). Although the vaccine virus is purified away from the cells, small amounts of animal cell proteins or DNA sometimes remain. The remaining amounts are so small that they are measured in nanograms (billionths of a gram) or picograms (trillionths of a gram). It is fair to say that we are all exposed to far greater quantities of nonhuman proteins or DNA when we eat food.

Gelatin

One animal product in vaccines, however, is present in fairly large quantities: gelatin (see "Do Vaccines Contain Products to Which People Could Be Allergic?"). Gelatin used in vaccines, derived from the skin and hooves of pigs, is highly purified and hydrolyzed (broken down by water) to make much smaller molecules than are found in nature. Unlike animal cell proteins and DNA, the amount of gelatin contained in vaccines isn't small. For example, the chickenpox (varicella) vaccine contains about 8 milligrams (thousandths of a gram) of gelatin. Some religious groups, such as Jewish people, Muslims, and Seventh Day Adventists follow dietary guidelines that oppose the ingestion of pig products. However, religious leaders from all three of these groups have sanctioned the use of gelatin-containing vaccines for several reasons. First, vaccines are injected, not ingested (only the rotavirus vaccine is ingested, and it doesn't contain gelatin). Second, the gelatin in vaccines is modified enough to render it sufficiently different from natural gelatin. Third, the benefits of receiving a vaccine outweigh adherence to the religion's dietary principles.

Reference

Institute for Vaccine Safety. "Religious Leaders Approval of Use of Vaccines Containing Porcine Gelatin." March 4, 2021.

DO VACCINES CONTAIN MICROCHIPS?

When COVID-19 vaccines first became available in December 2020, many conspiracy theories were spawned by antivaccine activists. One conspiracy theory centered on the notion that Bill Gates planned to inject everyone with microchips. In addition to the fact that Bill Gates does not work for or have decision-making power at any of the companies manufacturing COVID-19 vaccines, microchips, which are roughly the size of a grain of rice, are too large to fit through the bevel of a needle. Unfortunately, this false notion got more attention—and scared more people—than it ever should have, in part because fear spreads more easily than logic.

THE IMMUNE SYSTEM

HOW DOES THE IMMUNE SYSTEM PROCESS VACCINES?

Vaccines are typically injected into the arm or leg or, in the case of the rotavirus vaccine, squirted into the mouth. All vaccines, except for the COVID-19 mRNA vaccines, contain viral proteins or bacterial proteins or polysaccharides (which are the sugar coatings on the surface of bacteria). In the case of the mRNA vaccines, our cells make the viral proteins. The result after any type of vaccine is the same: our immune system springs into action. The vaccine proteins or polysaccharides are first taken up by specialized immune system cells called dendritic cells and macrophages, which begin to process them. The antigens (the parts of the vaccine that the immune system responds to) are then broken down into tiny fragments and placed on the surface of immune system cells. These "antigen-decorated" cells, known as antigen-presenting cells, then travel to the local lymph nodes. In the case of vaccines given in the arm, the local lymph nodes are under the arm. For those given in the thigh, the local lymph nodes are in the groin, and for those given by mouth, the local lymph nodes are just under the intestinal lining.

Once in the lymph nodes, the antigen-presenting cells activate other immune system cells, like B cells (which make antibodies) and T cells (which either help B cells make antibodies or kill virus-infected cells). The activation of these cells, as well as immune system signaling chemicals, composes the immune response against the vaccine. In the process, immunologic memory specific for the antigen delivered by the vaccine is also generated. So, the next time your body sees that antigen, it can respond faster and stronger.

HOW MUCH IMMUNITY CAN A VACCINE PROVIDE?

Some viral vaccines are so good that they can prevent even mild illness for decades following vaccination and eliminate the virus from the face of the earth. Others are good at protecting against serious disease but not as good at protecting against mild disease. The difference is determined by the incubation period of the disease, which is the time between exposure to a virus and the onset of symptoms.

If the incubation period is long (meaning a couple of weeks), as for smallpox and measles, then the disease can be eliminated. If the incubation period is short (meaning only a few days), as for influenza, rotavirus, and SARS-CoV-2 (the virus that causes COVID-19), then the virus is likely to circulate for centuries causing mild illness in most people and severe disease in some.

WHY DOES THE INCUBATION PERIOD OF A DISEASE
DETERMINE THE EFFECTIVENESS OF A VACCINE?

First, we need to understand a few things about how the immune system works, including differences in the immune response the first time our bodies see a pathogen (the specific cause of a disease, such as a bacterium or virus) as well as which parts of the immune system are required to prevent mild illness and which are required to prevent severe illness.

WHAT HAPPENS THE FIRST TIME OUR BODY SEES A PATHOGEN?

Our immune system has two parts: the innate and adaptive immune systems. The innate immune system is our first line of defense, and it includes things like physical barriers (e.g., skin, tear ducts, coughing, and vomiting) and chemical barriers (e.g., stomach acids, chemicals and mucus in the oral and genital tracts, and pus, which is collections of white blood cells and cellular debris). Our innate immune system does a fabulous job of keeping most pathogens from getting into our bloodstream and organs. But, when our external barriers are breached, the innate immune system activates our adaptive immune system.

The adaptive immune system is more strategic in its response—creating cells and proteins specific to the invading pathogen or antigen. The result of adaptive immune responses is antibodies, B cells, and T cells that are specific for only a single pathogen or antigen. The first time the adaptive immune response is activated against a pathogen is called the primary immune response because even though the immune response is specific, the immune system is just "learning" about the new pathogen. Along the way, it is also developing an important part of subsequent responses to the same pathogen: immunologic memory.

WHAT HAPPENS DURING REPEAT EXPOSURES TO A PATHOGEN?

After surviving the primary encounter with an antigen, some parts of the adaptive immune response linger. Antibodies produced during an immune response last for a short time, usually three to six months. However, memory B and T cells remain, circulating at low levels in the body, often for decades, to monitor for future encounters. If a person is exposed to the same pathogen again, these memory cells respond more quickly, making secondary, or memory, immune responses much more efficient than the primary immune response. Vaccination leverages the benefits of immunologic memory by intentionally introducing a primary infection in a controlled manner so that the individual develops immunologic memory without enduring the illness associated with a primary infection.

THE EFFECTIVENESS OF IMMUNOLOGIC MEMORY

It would be nice to think that once we have immunologic memory to a pathogen, we are set, but it's not quite that simple. For diseases with short incubation periods, like influenza, rotavirus, and COVID-19, symptoms begin *before* memory cells have had enough time to spring into action. The only way to prevent these symptoms, then, is to have antibodies present at the time of exposure. Since antibodies are short-lived (three to six months), people with immunologic memory, but without antibodies at the time of exposure, can suffer mild illness. Where mild infections occur only a few days after exposure, it takes much more time, about a couple of weeks, to develop severe disease. That's plenty of time for memory cells to have an effect, in most cases stopping the infection from becoming more severe. The differences between the roles and longevity of antibodies versus memory cells explain why protection against mild disease is short-lived while protection against severe disease is long-lived. Let's take a closer look.

The key determinant for protection against mild illness is the level of virus-specific antibodies that remain in the bloodstream at the time of exposure to the virus. The good news is that these antibodies are readily induced by both natural infection and vaccination. The bad news, as mentioned earlier, is that they don't last very long—usually three to six months—before they fade away. Therefore, for diseases with short incubation periods, protection against mild illness is always short-lived.

Protection against severe illness, on the other hand, can benefit from immunologic memory because in the time it takes for severe illness to develop, immunologic memory cells can expand, producing antibodies and other chemical signals that the immune system relies on to shut down the infection. Further, with each subsequent exposure to the pathogen, memory cells become more specialized in identifying it and thus more efficient.

THE IMPORTANCE OF THE INCUBATION PERIOD

If a person does not become infected with a virus, they cannot transmit it to others. However, as we've just seen, even when vaccination results in long-term protection from severe illness because of immunologic memory, a person can still experience mild illness if the disease has a short incubation period. During the first few days following exposure, while immunologic memory is ramping up, the virus can reproduce and cause symptoms. Since symptoms can be mild, or not felt at all (as in so-called asymptomatic infections), an infected individual can spread the virus to others during this period, which is one reason that it is not possible to eliminate diseases with short incubation periods. On the other hand, long incubation periods better position us for possible elimination of some diseases, like smallpox, polio, and measles.

IS HERD IMMUNITY REAL?

Herd immunity is real, but it is only one type of immunity from which people can benefit, so let's take a closer look. Three types of immunity are relevant to our discussion: active immunity, passive immunity, and herd immunity.

Active Immunity

Active immunity is the gold standard among the three types of immunity because it is immunity for a specific pathogen that has been generated by a person's own immune system. Active immunity can result from either infection or vaccination. Unfortunately, throughout life there are also times when people need to rely on immunity generated by others. This is where passive and herd immunity come in.

Passive Immunity

Passive immunity results when a person is protected using antibodies generated by someone else. These antibodies can be introduced in two ways: to an unborn child during pregnancy or by medical intervention. For example, newborns are typically protected against infections because of the presence of maternal antibodies that crossed the placenta before birth or from antibodies they consume in breast milk after birth.

Antivenom, often used to treat snake bites, is another example of passive immunity. During the COVID-19 pandemic, before vaccines were available, antibody-laden serum collected from people who had recovered from SARS-CoV-2 infection was used to treat some of the more severely ill people. And, a new treatment intended to protect babies from respiratory syncytial virus (RSV) during their first year or two of life, called nirsevimab, is also based on the concept of passive immunity, although here, the antibody is made in a laboratory, not another person.

Importantly, passive immunity is not as good as active immunity because although it provides antibodies that offer immediate protection, these antibodies are short-lived, and the individual does not have the opportunity to develop immunologic memory. As such, this type of immunity does not offer long-term protection.

Herd Immunity

Herd immunity is sometimes called community immunity because protection comes from being around others in one's community who are protected. Herd immunity works like this: If most people in a community (e.g., a house, a classroom, or a town) are immune to a pathogen, that pathogen will not have as many opportunities to spread through that community.

Conversely, if few people are immune, the pathogen has many opportunities to spread. Pathogens survive by spreading, so they excel at finding the weaknesses in a community's immunity. For some people, herd immunity is critically important because they rely on it for protection. This can be the case for several reasons:

- A person's immune system is weak because of a chronic health condition, a short-term illness, or a medical treatment such as chemotherapy.
- A person is too young to get a vaccine, such as a newborn.
- A person has a medical condition that precludes vaccination, such as a severe allergy to a vaccine ingredient.

At any given time, many people in a community rely on those around them for protection, and we all have family members who will need to rely on herd immunity at some point. If too many people opt out of vaccination because of safety concerns or religious or personal beliefs, the community will be less safe—not only for them but also for those who rely on the community for protection. In this way, vaccination decisions are different from other medical decisions: medical decisions most often affect only the person making them, but vaccine decisions affect a person's entire community.

Interestingly, studies have shown that in communities with weak herd immunity, even people immune from vaccination or previous infection are at greater risk of illness. This is because vaccines are not 100 percent effective, so some vaccinated people will still be susceptible to infection, and some previous infections, particularly mild ones, do not generate robust enough immunity to protect a person from all future encounters with that pathogen.

So, while herd immunity is helpful, and arguably necessary for some, it is not as foolproof as active immunity. The best-case scenario is to be protected by active immunity and to reside in a highly protected community.

The Role of the Pathogen in Herd Immunity

As mentioned, some vaccines can eliminate viruses from the world. Others can't (see "How Much Immunity Can a Vaccine Provide?").

Let's start with measles. In 2000, when about 95 percent of the population was immunized or had been previously infected, the United States eliminated measles. Those who couldn't be vaccinated, such as very young children and people with immune-compromising health conditions, were still protected. The herd protected them.

Rotavirus is different from measles. The rotavirus vaccine was introduced in 2006. Soon, more than 90 percent of babies were immunized. Consequently, severe disease, as measured by the number of hospitalizations from rotavirus-induced dehydration, was virtually eliminated. But because rotaviruses have a short incubation period, the virus could still cause mild or asymptomatic infections and be transmitted to others. Even though infections still occur in this scenario, the amount of virus produced during an infection in a vaccinated individual is typically much less than would be produced in an unvaccinated person (due to immunologic memory). This would still be considered herd immunity because vaccination slows the spread of the virus throughout a community and cases of severe disease decrease, but it is more difficult to protect people from mild infections caused by a pathogen of this type.

SARS-CoV-2 infections are like rotavirus infections. By early 2023, when about 95 percent of the population had been either naturally infected or immunized, the incidence of hospitalizations and deaths decreased dramatically. But the virus still circulated in the community, causing mild disease in many and severe disease in some. Some thought this meant that COVID-19 vaccines were not working, but the reality was that they were working exactly as they would be predicted to, based on the characteristics of the pathogen.

DID YOU KNOW?

One famous example of passive immunity involved the use of diphtheria antitoxin, a preparation of antibodies against the toxin produced by the bacterium that causes diphtheria. In 1925, before a diphtheria vaccine was available, an outbreak in Nome, Alaska, threatened the members of that community. The town's doctor did not have any diphtheria antitoxin, and the closest supply was a thousand miles away in Anchorage. But, because of the weather, the only way to get the antitoxin to the town was via train to Nenana and then via teams of dogs relaying it over the remaining seven hundred miles. The effort was dubbed "The Great Race of Mercy" taking five and a half days (half the time of the previous record), 150 dogs, and twenty mushers to complete. Balto, the lead dog of the team that arrived in Nome, became the most famous dog involved in this effort. The annual Iditarod race, still run today, commemorates this life-saving journey.

HOW DO WE KNOW THAT DIFFERENT VACCINES CAN BE GIVEN AT THE SAME TIME?

Before the Food and Drug Administration (FDA) will license a new vaccine, it must first be tested in concomitant-use studies in which the new vaccine is given with existing vaccines at the same time. The new vaccine must be shown not to interfere with the safety or immunogenicity (the immune response) of existing vaccines, and existing vaccines must be shown not to interfere with the safety or immunogenicity of the new vaccine. These studies take years to complete and cost millions of dollars. Because concomitant-use studies have been required for decades, hundreds of studies have been performed showing that children can safely be inoculated with multiple vaccines at the same time.

Reference

Orenstein, Walter A., Paul A. Offit, Kathryn M. Edwards, and Stanley A. Plotkin, eds. *Plotkin's Vaccines*, 8th ed. London: Elsevier, 2024.

CAN TOO MANY VACCINES OVERWHELM THE IMMUNE SYSTEM?

Today, young children get vaccines to prevent fifteen different diseases. That can mean as many as twenty-seven inoculations altogether and as many as five shots given at one time. It's difficult for a parent to watch this; they might wonder if it is too many. So, the question is perfectly reasonable and while the answer is no, the reasons why are worth understanding.

First, let's compare the number of immunological challenges in vaccines today with those in the past. In the 1980s, children received vaccines against seven diseases: measles, mumps, and rubella (combined as MMR vaccine); diphtheria, tetanus, and pertussis (combined as DTP vaccine); and polio. In the 1950s, children received vaccines against five diseases: diphtheria, tetanus, and pertussis (combined as DTP); polio; and smallpox. At the turn of the twentieth century, children received just one vaccine: smallpox. Most parents today would probably be surprised to learn that the number of immunological components contained in that one vaccine given a hundred years ago was greater than the number contained in all vaccines given to prevent fifteen diseases today.

To understand why, let's begin by defining terms. An immunological component, or antigen, is that part of a virus or bacterium that induces an immune response (like making specific antibodies). For viruses, immunological components consist of viral proteins; for bacteria, they consist of bacterial proteins or polysaccharides, which are complex sugars that surround the bacterial surface. The smallpox vaccine contained about two hundred proteins. The vaccines given to protect young children against fifteen diseases today contain a total of about 160 proteins. So, although there is no denying that fifteen vaccines are more than one, it's what's *in* the vaccines, not the number of vaccines, that counts. Fortunately, thanks to advances in protein chemistry, protein purification, and recombinant DNA technology, vaccines today are much purer (and consequently safer) than those used in the past.

Second, let's compare vaccines with other immunological challenges in the environment—challenges that are unseen but much greater than those in vaccines. The womb is sterile: no bacteria, no viruses, no parasites, no fungi. So, fetal immune systems aren't required to do much. But as the baby passes through the birth canal and enters the outside world, that changes quickly; the baby is immediately confronted with trillions of bacteria. These bacteria live on the lining of the nose, throat, skin, and intestines. Indeed, about ten times more bacteria live on the surface of our bodies (about one hundred trillion) than we have cells in our bodies (about ten trillion). And that's not the end of it: the food that children eat isn't sterile, nor is the air they inhale. Most bacteria have the capacity to invade the bloodstream and cause harm, and each bacterium contains between two thousand and six thousand immunological components. To prevent this from happening, babies' bodies make large quantities of antibodies every day. Grams of them. That's a tremendous commitment by the baby to make one type of protein (antibodies). In addition, soon after they're born, babies encounter a variety of viruses that can't be prevented by vaccines—like rhinoviruses (which cause the common cold), parainfluenza virus, adenovirus, norovirus, calicivirus, astrovirus, echovirus, coxsackie virus, human metapneumovirus, parechovirus, parvovirus, and enterovirus. And unlike vaccine viruses, which reproduce poorly or not at all, natural viruses reproduce thousands of times, causing an intense immune response. Studies have shown that healthy children experience between six and eight viral infections every year during their first few years of life. Vaccines don't prevent most of these.

Third, let's calculate the extent to which vaccines challenge the immune system. Exactly how many vaccines can a baby respond to? The best reasoned answer to this question comes from a paper written by two immunologists at the University of California San Diego, Mel Cohn and Rod Langman. Cohn and Langman focused on antibodies, an important component of the immune response induced by vaccines. Antibodies are made by B cells, each of which has the capacity to make antibodies against only one immunological unit, called an epitope. By calculating the number of B cells in the bloodstream, the average number of epitopes contained in a vaccine, and the rapidity with which a critical quantity of antibodies could be made, we know that a baby could theoretically respond to *one hundred thousand* vaccines at one time.

Of course, we're not saying that babies should get a hundred thousand vaccines at once. We're saying only that they could handle it. Indeed, given that babies are constantly confronted with trillions of bacteria and that each bacterium contains thousands of immunological components, this shouldn't be surprising. In a sense, babies are responding to such an assault every day.

Fourth, let's examine how well newborns respond to vaccines by looking at the hepatitis B vaccine (see the section titled "Hepatitis B"). Babies born to mothers infected with hepatitis B virus are at high risk of not only being infected with the virus but also developing cirrhosis (chronic liver damage) or liver cancer. The greatest risk of infection and long-term problems comes at the time of delivery. Hepatitis B virus is present in large quantities in the blood of infected people. So, when passing through the bloody birth canal of an infected mother, a baby encounters an incredible amount of hepatitis B virus. Each milliliter (about one-fifth of a teaspoon) of blood from someone infected with hepatitis B contains roughly one billion infectious viruses, and the birth process exposes a baby to a lot of blood. So, it's no wonder that almost all children born to infected mothers contract the disease.

The hepatitis B vaccine is given shortly after birth, and in cases where the baby was exposed to the virus during delivery, studies have shown that about 80 percent of babies are protected against infection after just one dose of hepatitis B vaccine, which contains only 20 micrograms (millionths of a gram) of one protein from the virus. That's amazing. And it speaks to the remarkable resiliency and strength of the newborn's immune system. But it shouldn't be surprising. Given the natural onslaught from challenges in the environment, babies must be ready to respond to a tremendous microbial onslaught the minute they are born if they are to survive.

Indeed, babies are typically exposed to diseases like *Haemophilus influenzae* type b (Hib), pneumococcus, rotavirus, and pertussis (whooping cough) early in life. If they are to avoid these diseases, they need to develop an immune response quickly. While maternal antibodies directed against many of these infections are passed on to babies while still in the womb, these antibodies eventually fade away, leaving the child vulnerable (this is an example of *passive immunity*). That's why vaccines against Hib, pneumococcus, rotavirus, and pertussis are given at two, four, and six months of age, so when passive immunity fades, the child will have developed their own immunity, which is called *active immunity*. For more on active and passive immunity, see "Is Herd Immunity Real?"

References

Cohn, Melvin, and Rodney E. Langman. "The Protecton: The Unit of Humoral Immunity Selected by Evolution." *Immunological Reviews* 115 (1990): 11–147.

Dingle, John H., George F. Badger, and William S. Jordan. *Illness in the Home: A Study of 25,000 Illnesses in a Group of Cleveland Families*. Cleveland: Press of Western Reserve University, 1964.

Offit, Paul A., Jessica Quarles, Michael A. Gerber, et al. "Addressing Parents' Concerns: Do Multiple Vaccines Overwhelm or Weaken the Infant's Immune System?" *Pediatrics* 109, no. 1 (2002): 124–29.

CAN TOO MANY VACCINES WEAKEN THE IMMUNE SYSTEM?

One way to answer this question is to determine whether vaccinated children are at greater risk of infections not prevented by vaccines than those who are unvaccinated—in other words, whether vaccines weaken the immune systems of vaccinated children to the extent that they can't respond effectively to other viruses or bacteria. In fact, the opposite appears to be true. In Germany, a study of about five hundred children found that those who had received immunizations against diphtheria, pertussis, tetanus, Hib, and polio within the first three months of life had *fewer* infections with viruses and bacteria *not* prevented by those vaccines than unvaccinated children. Other studies have confirmed this observation.

Indeed, one can argue that vaccines strengthen the immune system by not only providing immunity to specific viruses and bacteria but also preventing secondary infections. A secondary infection is an infection that occurs after an initial infection caused by another pathogen, known as the primary infection, has weakened a person's immune system. For example, people with pneumonia caused by pneumococcus are more likely to have had a recent influenza infection. Therefore, preventing influenza will, to some extent, also prevent pneumococcal pneumonia. Similarly, having had chickenpox increases one's susceptibility to diseases such as necrotizing fasciitis (in which bacteria eat through muscles and tendons), pyomyositis (in which muscles liquefy because of intense inflammation), toxic shock syndrome (which causes dangerously low blood pressure), and bacteremia (in which bacteria invade the bloodstream). All these diseases are caused by group A β-hemolytic *streptococci*, often referred to in the popular press as "flesh-eating bacteria." Therefore, by preventing chickenpox, we can also prevent some serious strep infections.

References

Davidson, Michael, William Letson, Joel I. Ward, et al. "DTP Immunization and Susceptibility to Infectious Diseases: Is There a

Relationship?" *American Journal of Diseases of Children* 145, no. 7 (1991): 750–54.

Laupland, Kevin B., H. Dele Davies, Donald E. Low, et al. "Invasive Group A Streptococcal Disease in Children and Association with Varicella-Zoster Virus Infection." *Pediatrics* 105, no. 5 (2000): e60.

O'Brien, Katherine L., M. Ingre Walters, Jonathan Sellman, et al. "Severe Pneumococcal Pneumonia in Previously Healthy Children: The Role of Preceding Influenza Infection." *Clinical Infectious Diseases* 30, no. 5 (2000): 784–89.

Otto, S., B. Mahner, I. Kadow, et al. "General Non-specific Morbidity Is Reduced After Vaccination Within the Third Month of Life—The Greifswald Study." *Journal of Infection* 41, no. 2 (2000): 172–75.

Storsaeter, Jann, Patrick Olin, Berit Renemar, et al. "Mortality and Morbidity from Invasive Bacterial Infections During a Clinical Trial of Acellular Pertussis Vaccines in Sweden." *Pediatric Infectious Disease Journal* 7, no. 9 (1988): 637–45.

ARE BABIES TOO YOUNG TO GET VACCINATED?

The moment babies enter the world, they are bombarded by bacteria and viruses. We are born when we are ready to meet these challenges to our immune system. Babies in the first few weeks of life are somewhat less capable of fending off bacterial infections because one type of white blood cell (called neutrophils) is still maturing. Children in the first two years of life also don't make very good immune responses to the complex sugar coating on the surface of bacteria (polysaccharide coating). For several years, this hindered our ability to protect children from some potentially severe bacterial infections. But researchers eventually got around this problem with the pneumococcal and Hib vaccines by linking the polysaccharide to a harmless protein in what are called conjugated vaccines.

The hepatitis B vaccine, which is given at birth, induces an excellent immune response. And many vaccines given at two, four, and six months of age also induce an excellent immune response. That's fortunate because many of these pathogens, like rotavirus, pneumococcus, and Hib cause disease in children between six and twenty-four months of age. Children must be fully immune to prevent such diseases. This is the main reason that babies get so many vaccines in the first few months of life. The timing of vaccinations in the immunization schedule is intentionally designed to ensure that babies are immune to certain diseases by the time they are most likely to be susceptible and exposed. For this reason, delaying or spacing out vaccinations is not without risk.

ISN'T IT BETTER TO BE NATURALLY INFECTED THAN IMMUNIZED?

For the most part, the immune response following natural infection is better than that induced by immunization. Whereas a single natural infection often induces protective immunity, it often takes several—sometimes as many as five—doses of a vaccine to induce protection. But natural infection occasionally comes with a high price: paralysis caused by polio, bloodstream infections caused by Hib, severe pneumonia caused by pneumococcus, permanent birth defects caused by rubella, and cancer caused by human papillomavirus (HPV), to name a few. So, although it might take a few doses of a vaccine to protect against natural infection, it's worth it.

Interestingly, some vaccines induce immune responses that are better than those from natural infection. The HPV vaccine, because it contains a highly purified version of one important protein of the virus, induces antibody levels much higher than those found after natural infection. Tetanus vaccine is another example. Tetanus bacteria make a toxin that causes severe muscle contractions (that's why the disease is occasionally referred to as lockjaw). This toxin is so potent that the amount required to cause disease is less than that which induces an immune response. For this reason, people infected with tetanus are still recommended to receive the tetanus vaccine.

Other examples of vaccines that induce immune responses better than natural infection are Hib and pneumococcal vaccines.

As a rule, children less than two years old make excellent immune responses to viruses, but they're not quite as good at making immune responses to certain bacteria: specifically, those that have complex sugar coatings called polysaccharides. Both Hib and pneumococcus have polysaccharides on their surfaces. If children are to be protected against these bacteria, they need to make an immune response to these polysaccharides, but they're unable to. So even if children survive meningitis, bloodstream infection, or pneumonia caused by Hib (see the section on *Haemophilus influenzae* type b), they're still recommended to receive the Hib vaccine.

Reference

Orenstein, Walter A., Paul A. Offit, Kathryn M. Edwards, and Stanley A. Plotkin, eds. *Plotkin's Vaccines*, 8th ed. London: Elsevier, 2024.

PRACTICAL CONSIDERATIONS

ARE VACCINES FREE?

Insurance companies typically pay for recommended vaccines. For children who are uninsured or underinsured, the Vaccines for Children (VFC) Program (https://www.cdc.gov/vaccines/programs/vfc/parents/index.html) pays for vaccines. For adults who are uninsured or underinsured, public health departments will sometimes cover the cost of certain vaccines, or they may know of programs in the area that will do so.

Vaccines for international travel may not be covered by insurance or government programs, so it's a good idea to look into which vaccines may be needed well in advance. Seek advice from travel clinics when possible because they often stock these types of vaccines, and they can also provide information about how to prepare for and stay healthy during travel as well as what to watch for when you return.

HOW DO I DEAL WITH A FEAR OF SHOTS?

Many children are afraid to go to the doctor's office when they know it's time to get shots. However, some techniques can help them through this occasionally frightening experience.

Gina French and her colleagues at the Children's Hospital of Columbus, Ohio, published a study evaluating the capacity of breathing techniques to ease the pain of vaccines called "Blowing Away Shot Pain." French studied 150 children between four and seven years of age who were about to be immunized. Half the children were treated as usual. The other half were told, "I know a trick that might make it easier. It is something that children who get lots of shots use. When it is time for the shot, you should take a deep breath and blow and blow and blow until I tell you to stop." These children were then asked to practice this technique with the investigator. After the shots were given, the children were asked to evaluate their pain on a scale from "no pain at all" to "the worst pain in the world." Children who had been coached on the breathing technique rated their pain as significantly less than those who hadn't.

Children are not the only ones with a fear of needles and vaccines. The CARD System (Comfort Ask Relax Distract), developed in Canada, offers evidence-based techniques to help people of any age feel more comfortable and relaxed when receiving a vaccination. The system offers tips about distraction techniques and questions for vaccine recipients to ask as well as information about establishing a calming environment and approaches to giving vaccines for healthcare providers. While most studies of CARD have been completed in school-aged children, the system has also been evaluated at mass vaccination clinics and in community pharmacies, demonstrating improvements in the vaccination experience across age groups and settings. The CARD System resources for children, adults, caregivers, and health care providers can be found at https://www.aboutkidshealth .ca/card/.

References

French, Gina M., Eileen C. Painter, and Daniel L. Coury. "Blowing Away Shot Pain: A Technique for Pain Management During Immunization." *Pediatrics* 93, no. 3 (1994): 384–88.

Taddio, Anna, Victoria Gudzak, Marlene Jantzi, et al. "Impact of the CARD (Comfort Ask Relax Distract) System on School-Based Vaccinations: A Cluster Randomized Trial." *Vaccine* 40, no. 19 (2022):2802–9.

Taddio, Anna, James Morrison, Victoria Gudzak, et al. "CARD (Comfort Ask Relax Distract) for Community Pharmacy Vaccinations in Children: Effect on Immunization Stress-Related Responses and Satisfaction." *Canadian Pharmacists Journal* 156, no. S1 (2023): 27S–35S.

Tetui, Moses, Kelly Grindrod, Nancy Waite, et al. "Integrating the CARD (Comfort Ask Relax Distract) System in a Mass Vaccination Clinic to Improve the Experience of Individuals During COVID-19 Vaccination: A Pre-Post Implementation Study." *Human Vaccines & Immunotherapeutics* 18, no. 5 (2022): 2089500.

WHAT CAN I DO TO MAKE VACCINATIONS LESS STRESSFUL?

Whether you're taking a member of your family for a vaccination or getting your own, there are several things you can do before, during and after the appointment to make the visit less stressful (also check "How Do I Deal with a Fear of Shots?").

Before the visit:

- Find out which vaccines are due.
- Bring the person's immunization record.
- Write down any questions you have.
- Bring along a favorite book, electronic game, toy, or blanket, depending on the age of the person receiving the vaccination.

During the visit:

- Read the Vaccine Information Statements (VISs) that are available in doctors' offices. If you are not provided with these, ask an office staff member.
- Ask the healthcare team any questions you have about vaccines before they bring them into the room.

- If your infant or young child is getting immunized, hold them on your lap. Preteens, teens, and adults should be seated or lying down during immunizations.
- If you are there supporting a family member, talk reassuringly, make eye contact, smile, and offer physical comfort, such as holding an older person's hand or cuddling a young child before and immediately following the shots. It's important to realize that if you demonstrate apprehension, your family member will likely pick up on that and react accordingly, particularly young children who rely on their parents and caregivers for comfort.

After the visit:

- If the area where the shot was given is red, tender, or swollen, apply a cool, wet cloth or ice to the area.
- Some people develop fever following vaccination, which is an indication that their body is responding to the vaccine. As such, treating fever after vaccination is not typically recommended, but if you have questions, talk with your health care provider. Importantly, if a pregnant person develops a fever following vaccination, it should be treated since a fever can harm the unborn baby.
- Ensure that the vaccinated individual drinks plenty of fluids and realize that they may be less interested in food during the next 24 hours.
- Watch for signs of severe reactions, such as prolonged fever, unusual behavior, or new, severe, or unexpected symptoms. If you have any concerns, call the health care provider where the vaccine was administered for guidance.

Most reactions to vaccines are mild. However, if someone experiences a more severe reaction, they should report it to the Vaccine Adverse Event Reporting System (VAERS): http://vaers.hhs.gov /index. Anyone can submit a report to VAERS.

WHAT SHOULD I EXPECT TO FEEL AFTER A VACCINATION? WHAT SHOULD I WATCH OUT FOR?

Vaccines sometimes cause a knot, or hard area, at the site of inoculation, usually as a result of a vaccine adjuvant. This knot usually goes away in a few days, but if it doesn't, it would be reasonable to have your health care provider look at it.

Vaccines induce an immune response. Some of the proteins made by the immune system in response to a vaccine (with names like cytokines and interferons) can themselves cause symptoms, like muscle aches, joint pain, joint stiffness, headache, and fever. These symptoms are normal and should go away within a few days. However, if you're not sure if a reaction is normal or if you have concerns about the severity or length of symptoms, contact the health care provider where the vaccine was given.

SHOULD I TREAT A FEVER THAT DEVELOPS AFTER VACCINATION?

For all mammalian species (including humans), fever is part of the immune response. We develop a fever because our immune system works better at a higher temperature than at normal body temperature. Indeed, some studies have shown that giving fever-reducing medications (called antipyretics) before or immediately after vaccination can reduce the immune response, and indeed, many studies have shown that treating fever can prolong or worsen a variety of bacterial and viral illnesses by weakening the immune response.

So, unless you or your family member are very uncomfortable, you should try to embrace the day or two of low-grade fever following vaccination.

As mentioned, one exception when it comes to treating fevers is during pregnancy. Pregnant people who develop fever following vaccination should be treated as maternal fever can harm the unborn baby.

Reference

Offit, Paul A. *Overkill: When Modern Medicine Goes Too Far.* New York: Harper, 2020.

WHO SHOULD NOT GET VACCINES?

Some people can't be vaccinated because they are unable to make an adequate immune response. These people fall into four groups: those receiving immune-suppressive drugs for cancer, a rheumatological condition, or severe asthma; those born with an immune deficiency; those chronically infected with an immunosuppressive virus (specifically, human immunodeficiency virus [HIV], the cause of AIDS); and those who are chronically ill and relatively malnourished.

No simple formula is available to determine who should or should not get vaccines in these situations. The answer depends on the degree of immune suppression, which is best determined by the person's physician. As a rule, inactivated vaccines (like the COVID-19; diphtheria, tetanus, pertussis; hepatitis A; hepatitis B; Hib; human papillomavirus [HPV]; influenza [the shot]; meningococcus; mpox; pneumococcus; polio; respiratory syncytial virus [RSV]; and shingles vaccines) can be given safely. However, for some people who are immune suppressed, these vaccines might not induce an adequate immune response.

Live, weakened (attenuated) viral vaccines (like chickenpox; influenza [the nasal spray]; measles, mumps, rubella [MMR]; and rotavirus vaccines) are a different story. Because these vaccine viruses can replicate, and because replication might not be controllable in those who cannot develop an adequate immune response, these vaccines can be dangerous. So, whereas inactivated or non-live viral or bacterial vaccines may not be given because they might be ineffective, live, weakened viral vaccines should *not* be given because they might be unsafe.

The bottom line is that your doctor, in concert with the oncologist, rheumatologist, allergist, or whoever is primarily responsible for giving immune-suppressive drugs, needs to decide whether the degree of immune suppression precludes giving inactivated vaccines, live weakened vaccines, or both. Because people who are immune compromised are at greater risk of developing severe infections caused by vaccine-preventable diseases, the people around them should be fully vaccinated, particularly those living in the home.

Reference

Centers for Disease Control and Prevention. "General Recommendations on Immunization: Recommendations of the Advisory Committee on Immunization Practices." *Morbidity and Mortality Weekly Report* 55 (2006): 24–29.

HOW CAN I PROTECT MY BABY BEFORE THEY ARE OLD ENOUGH TO BE VACCINATED?

While in the womb, babies are in a sterile environment. Once they enter the world, they encounter many different bacteria and viruses in the first few years of life. Although babies' immune systems can protect them to some degree and they also benefit from maternal antibodies that crossed the placenta and are in breast milk, they are still fairly vulnerable to infection, especially in the first couple of months of life. For these reasons, parents should try to limit their young infants' contact with large numbers of people (e.g., such as passing a new baby around to multiple people during a family gathering) and ask people to refrain from visiting if they are ill. Asking people to wash their hands before holding the baby and limiting touches and kisses on the face can also help, particularly if there are young children around the baby. Generally, however, there is no hard-and-fast rule on this; it's mostly a matter of common sense and what the parents are comfortable with.

If you are a visitor, it is important to respect the wishes of the parents and understand that they are just trying to protect their new baby.

CAN I GET VACCINATED IF I'M ILL?

Some parents might worry that children with minor illnesses—such as those causing runny nose, itchy eyes, fever, vomiting, or diarrhea—might not be able to make an adequate immune response to vaccines or might be more likely to experience vaccine side effects. The good news is that researchers have shown that immune responses and side effects following vaccination are

the same in both healthy children and children with a mild illness. Therefore, children with mild illnesses can still receive all
routinely recommended vaccines on schedule.

Studies of vaccines in children with severe infections (such as
pneumonia, bloodstream infection, or meningitis) are lacking.
Although a delay in vaccination in such cases is recommended, it's
not because children are unlikely to make an adequate immune
response. Rather, it's to avoid confusing a side effect to the vaccine with a symptom of the illness.

The same rules apply for older children and adults.

References

Dennehy, Penelope H., Georges Peter, and Cheryl L. Saracen. "Sero-
conversion Rates to Combined Measles-Mumps-Rubella-Varicella
Vaccine of Children with Upper Respiratory Tract Infection."
Pediatrics 94, no. 4 (1994): 514–16.

Halsey, Neal A., Reginald Boulos, Frantz Mode, et al. "Response to
Measles Vaccine in Haitian Infants 6 to 12 Months Old: Influence
of Maternal Antibodies, Malnutrition, and Concurrent Illness."
New England Journal of Medicine 313, no. 9 (1985): 544–49.

King, Gail E., Lauri E. Markowitz, Janet Heath, et al. "Antibody
Response to Measles-Mumps-Rubella Vaccine of Children with
Mild Illness at the Time of Vaccination." *Journal of the American
Medical Association* 275, no. 9 (1996): 704–7.

Ndikuyeze, Andre, Alvaro Munoz, John Stewart, et al. "Immunogenicity and Safety of Measles Vaccine in Ill African Children."
International Journal of Epidemiology 17, no. 2 (1988): 448–55.

Ratnam, Samuel, Roy West, and Veeresh Gadag. "Measles and Rubella
Antibody Response After Measles-Mumps-Rubella Vaccination in
Children with Afebrile Upper Respiratory Tract Infection." *Journal
of Pediatrics* 127, no. 3 (1995): 432–34.

CAN I VACCINATE MY PREMATURE BABY?

The length of time from conception to birth is about forty weeks.
But some children are born earlier. Those born before thirty-seven

weeks of gestation are considered premature. Parents of these infants often wonder whether, because of their early birth and small size, premature babies can adequately respond to vaccines designed for more developed infants and whether these vaccines are safe. Fortunately, studies have shown that all infants, independent of the degree of prematurity and weight, can be immunized according to their chronological age. In other words, if a baby is born one month prematurely, you don't have to wait until they are three months old to give a vaccine designed for two-month-olds. You can give the vaccine when the baby is two months old.

There is, however, one exception to this rule: hepatitis B vaccine. Premature babies who weigh less than 2,000 grams (about 4.5 pounds) do not make an adequate immune response to the hepatitis B vaccine given at birth. For them, the first dose of the hepatitis B vaccine should be delayed until one month of age.

References

Bernbaum, Judy C., Andrea Daft, Robert Anolik, et al. "Response of Preterm Infants to Diphtheria-Tetanus-Pertussis Immunizations." *Journal of Pediatrics* 107, no. 2 (1985): 184–88.

Kim, Susan C., Esther K. Chung, Richard L. Hodinka, et al. "Immunogenicity of Hepatitis B Vaccine in Preterm Infants." *Pediatrics* 99, no. 4 (1997): 534–36.

Koblin, B. A., T. R. Townsend, A. Munoz, et al. "Response of Preterm Infants to Diphtheria-Tetanus-Pertussis Vaccine." *Pediatric Infectious Disease Journal* 7, no. 10 (1988): 704–11.

Lau, Yu-Lung, Alfred Y. C. Tam, K. W. Ng, et al. "Response of Preterm Infants to Hepatitis B Vaccine." *Journal of Pediatrics* 121, no. 6 (1992): 962–65.

Losonsky, Genevieve A., Steven S. Wasserman, Ina Stephens, et al. "Hepatitis B Vaccination of Premature Infants: A Reassessment of Current Recommendations for Delayed Immunization." *Pediatrics* 103, no. 2 (1999): e14.

Omenaca, Felix, José Garcia-Sicilia, Pilar García-Corbeira, et al. "Response of Preterm Newborns to Immunization with Hexavalent

Diphtheria-Tetanus-Acellular Pertussis-Hepatitis B Virus-Inactivated Polio and *Haemophilus Influenzae* Type b Vaccine: First Experiences and Solutions to a Serious and Sensitive Issue." *Pediatrics* 116, no. 6 (2005): 1292–98.

Patel, Daksha M., Joyce Butler, Sandor Feldman, et al. "Immunogenicity of Hepatitis B Vaccine in Healthy Very Low Birth Weight Infants." *Journal of Pediatrics* 131, no. 4 (1997): 641–43.

Saari, T., AAP Committee on Infectious Diseases. "Immunization of Preterm and Low Birthweight Infants." *Pediatrics* 112 (2003): 193–198.

Shinefield, Henry, Steven Black, Paula Ray, et al. "Efficacy, Immunogenicity and Safety of Heptavalent Pneumococcal Conjugate Vaccine in Low Birth Weight and Preterm Infants." *Pediatric Infectious Disease Journal* 21, no. 3 (2002): 182–86.

Smolen, Paul, Regina Bland, Eric Heiligenstein, et al. "Antibody Response to Oral Polio Vaccine in Premature Infants." *Journal of Pediatrics* 103, no. 6 (1983): 917–19.

CAN I GET VACCINATED IF I'M TAKING STEROIDS?

Steroids are given for common conditions like asthma and reactions to poison ivy; they can also be used as immune-suppressive therapy following an organ or bone marrow transplant or as chemotherapy for cancer. Because steroids can significantly weaken the immune system, people often ask whether it is safe to give vaccines when someone is taking steroids.

The answer is yes and no. For those using steroid creams or sprays, vaccines can be given safely. Vaccines are also safe for those who have been taking steroids by mouth for less than two weeks. However, individuals who have received high doses of steroids for more than two weeks should *not* receive live, weakened viral vaccines, such as the chickenpox, MMR, nasal-spray influenza, and rotavirus vaccines. High doses of steroids can decrease a person's ability to eliminate vaccine viruses from the body, as well as their ability to make an adequate immune response to vaccination.

People can usually receive live, weakened viral vaccines one month after discontinuing immune-suppressive doses of steroids. Although inactivated or non-live vaccines (like COVID-19; diphtheria, tetanus, pertussis; hepatitis A; hepatitis B; Hib; HPV; influenza [the shot]; meningococcus; mpox; pneumococcus; polio; shingles; and RSV vaccines) can be given safely, it is better to postpone vaccination until at least one month after discontinuing immune-suppressive doses of steroids to ensure an adequate immune response.

Reference

Centers for Disease Control and Prevention. "General Recommendations on Immunization: Recommendations of the Advisory Committee on Immunization Practices." *Morbidity and Mortality Weekly Report* 55 (2006): 29.

CAN I GET VACCINATED IF I'M TAKING ANTIBIOTICS?

Yes. Antibiotics do not interfere with the effectiveness of vaccines, nor do they make any vaccine less safe.

CAN I GET VACCINATED IF I'M TAKING MEDICATIONS KNOWN AS BIOLOGICS?

Biologics are medications derived from living organisms that work by interacting with the immune system to treat diseases, particularly diseases that are the result of chronic conditions resulting from ongoing inflammatory responses of the immune system, like autoimmune diseases. Whether someone taking a biologic can be vaccinated depends on the specific biologic that they are taking. Some biologics interfere with the effectiveness of vaccines; others don't. If you're taking a biologic, check with your health care provider to see whether you are recommended to receive a specific vaccine.

To find out more about biologics and vaccines, see "Vaccines and Biologics: What You Should Know" from the Vaccine

Education Center at Children's Hospital of Philadelphia: https:// media.chop.edu/data/files/pdfs/vaccines-biologics.pdf.

CAN I GET VACCINATED IF I'M BEING TREATED FOR CANCER?

Whether someone undergoing treatment for cancer can get vaccinated depends on the type of drugs being administered to treat the cancer and where they are in the course of therapy (e.g., induction or maintenance phase). Talk with your health care provider to see if you can safely receive a vaccine or if you have any questions about vaccination.

CAN I GET VACCINATED IF I HAD OR WILL BE HAVING AN ORGAN TRANSPLANT?

Whether a person who has or will be undergoing an organ transplant can get vaccinated depends on the types of drugs being given to suppress the immune response to the transplanted organ and where they are in the transplant process. Talk with your health care provider to make sure that you can receive a vaccine safely and effectively.

CAN I GET VACCINATED IF I'M PREGNANT OR BREASTFEEDING?

Some vaccines can be given during pregnancy, and some can't; however, all vaccines can be given to someone who is breastfeeding.

All inactivated vaccines can be given during pregnancy. These include inactivated whole-virus vaccines (hepatitis A, influenza [the shot], and polio), vaccines that contain purified bacterial proteins (Tdap), vaccines that contain single viral proteins (COVID-19 [Novavax], hepatitis B, and HPV), and vaccines that contain complex sugars (polysaccharides) of bacteria (meningococcus and pneumococcus).

Live, weakened viral vaccines—specifically, the chickenpox, nasal-spray influenza, and MMR vaccines—should not be given during pregnancy. This isn't because these vaccines have been shown to be harmful; it's only because there is a theoretical risk of harm. A good example is the rubella vaccine. It is estimated that about 85 of 100 pregnant people naturally infected with rubella virus during the first trimester will deliver babies with permanent birth defects involving the eyes, ears, and heart. So, it would stand to reason that the rubella vaccine could do the same thing. But the rubella vaccine has been inadvertently administered to thousands of people during the first trimester of pregnancy and hasn't caused harm to their unborn children. That's because the vaccine virus is much weaker than the natural virus. For this reason, pregnant people who have mistakenly received rubella vaccine during the first trimester are counseled to continue their pregnancies.

Another example is the chickenpox vaccine. Chickenpox isn't nearly as risky as rubella when it comes to the potential for harming an unborn child, but natural chickenpox virus can cause birth defects. About 2 of 100 people infected with chickenpox virus during their pregnancy will deliver babies with shortened, deformed limbs and heads that are much smaller than normal. But, as with rubella vaccine, the chickenpox vaccine, when inadvertently administered during pregnancy, doesn't cause harm.

DID YOU KNOW?

The only vaccine that has ever been shown to harm a fetus if given during pregnancy is the smallpox vaccine. While smallpox has been eliminated from the world, other orthopoxviruses, like mpox, have resulted in the use of orthopoxvirus vaccines, including a live, weakened vaccine called ACAM2000, which should not be introduced during pregnancy or if the recipient cannot isolate from a pregnant household contact. A newer option, JYN-NEOS, does not replicate, so it offers alternatives if needed. Talk to a healthcare professional if you have questions.

Some vaccines are specifically recommended because of pregnancy. One important example is the influenza vaccine. Research has shown that pregnant women are six times more likely to be hospitalized and die from severe pneumonia caused by influenza virus than are those of the same age who aren't pregnant. In part, that's because as the baby grows, it presses against the lungs, making it more difficult to take deep breaths. Another reason that pregnant people are at higher risk of severe influenza infection is because their immune responses aren't as strong as those of their nonpregnant counterparts. During pregnancy, changes to the immune system prevent the developing baby, which has a different genetic makeup, from being identified as "foreign" and attacked by the pregnant person's immune system.

The COVID-19 vaccine is also recommended during pregnancy to protect the mother, who is at greater risk of developing severe disease if infected, as well as the child, who will acquire immunity from the mother that will last for the first six months of life. Women infected with SARS-CoV-2 virus during pregnancy are more likely to be hospitalized and require intensive care than women of the same age who aren't pregnant.

The Tdap vaccine, which protects against three infections, one of which is pertussis (whooping cough), is recommended for pregnant people between twenty-seven and thirty-six weeks of gestation during *every* pregnancy. Although a pregnant person can benefit from enhanced protection against pertussis, the main reason for this vaccination to be given during pregnancy is to protect the baby in the first few months of life—when they're most susceptible to pertussis and before they've had their own vaccinations against the disease, which can be deadly for young infants.

In October 2023, an RSV vaccine (Abrysvo) was approved and recommended for use between thirty-two and thirty-six weeks of pregnancy for those who will deliver during RSV season. The purpose of this vaccine is to generate antibodies that will be transferred to the unborn baby (via passive immunity) to protect them in their first months of life. In clinical trials testing this vaccine during pregnancy, those who were vaccinated were slightly more prone to preterm delivery compared with those who did not get the vaccine. For this reason, scientists and public health officials will continue to monitor this vaccine as more doses are given during pregnancy to determine whether this observation is confirmed as being causally associated. If you're wondering about getting this vaccine during pregnancy, talk with your health care provider to get the latest information.

DID YOU KNOW?

During the novel H1N1 influenza (swine flu) pandemic of 2009–2010, pregnant women were considered one of the highest-risk groups, so they were among the first to be vaccinated once vaccine became available.

References

Centers for Disease Control and Prevention. "COVID-19 Vaccines While Pregnant or Breastfeeding." Last updated November 3, 2023. https://www.cdc.gov/coronavirus/2019-ncov/vaccines/recommendations/pregnancy.html#:~:text=Recent%20data%20show%20that%20completing,hospitalization%20due%20to%20COVID%2D19.
Centers for Disease Control and Prevention. "General Recommendations on Immunization: Recommendations of the Advisory Committee on Immunization Practices." *Morbidity and Mortality Weekly Report* 55 (2006): 32–33.

SHOULD I VACCINATE MY CHILD IF I'M BREASTFEEDING?

Breastfeeding does not interfere with a baby's immune response to vaccines. Therefore, all breastfed infants can be immunized according to the normal schedule.

Some mothers also wonder whether they can receive vaccines while breastfeeding. Vaccines taken by a breastfeeding mother do not interfere with a baby's immune response to vaccines. Likewise getting vaccinated during the period a person is breastfeeding does not affect a vaccine's safety. Although live, weakened viral vaccines, like rubella vaccine, can multiply in the mother's body and consequently be excreted in breast milk, the vaccine virus is so weakened that it cannot harm the baby.

References

Bohlke, Kari, Karin Galil, Lisa A. Jackson, et al. "Postpartum Varicella Vaccination: Is the Vaccine Virus Excreted in Breast Milk?" *Obstetrics and Gynecology* 102, no. 5 (2003): 970–77.

Hahn-Zoric, M., F. Fulconis, I. Minoli, et al. "Antibody Responses to Parenteral and Oral Vaccines Are Impaired by Conventional and Low Protein Formulas as Compared to Breast Feeding." *Acta Paediatrica Scandanavica* 79, no. 12 (1990) 1137–42.

Kim-Farley, Robert, Edward Brink, Walter Orenstein, and Kenneth Bart. "Vaccination and Breast-Feeding." *Journal of the American Medical Association* 248, no. 19 (1982): 2451–52.

Krogh, V., L. C. Duffy, D. Wong, et al. "Postpartum Immunization with Rubella Virus Vaccine and Antibody Response in Breast-Feeding Infants." *Journal of Laboratory and Clinical Medicine* 113, no. 6 (1989): 695–99.

Patriarca, Peter A., Peter F. Wright, and T. Jacob John. "Factors Affecting the Immunogenicity of Oral Poliovirus Vaccine in Developing Countries: Review." *Review of Infectious Diseases* 13, no. 5 (1991): 926–39.

Pickering, Larry K., Dan M. Granoff, Julie Reed Erickson, et al. "Modulation of the Immune System by Human Milk and Infant Formula Containing Nucleotides." *Pediatrics* 101, no. 2 (1998): 242–49.

IS AN EXTRA DOSE OF VACCINE HARMFUL?

The vaccine schedule is busy. In the first few years of life, children are recommended to receive several inoculations, some of which are given at the same time. Also, many combination vaccines are available and often differ from one doctor's office to the next. Unfortunately, this complexity means that mistakes are occasionally made. In some cases, a child might receive an extra dose of vaccine. When this happens, parents of these children wonder whether the extra dose is harmful. While an extra shot may cause pain, redness, tenderness, or swelling at the injection site, the child is not more likely to suffer worse side effects. That's because the child has already started to make an immune response to the vaccine virus.

For example, suppose that a child who receives MMR vaccine develops a mild measles rash about a week later. This is an uncommon reaction that happens when measles vaccine virus travels to the skin. A parent could reasonably ask whether a child who develops a rash after the first dose of vaccine is more likely to develop a rash after the second dose. The answer is probably not because the child makes an immune response after the first dose. So, when give a second dose, the child has already developed some antibodies that limit the vaccine virus's ability to reproduce and travel to the skin.

Children who receive an extra dose of vaccine usually develop a boost in their immune response.

The same is generally true for adults who get an extra dose of vaccine. For example, someone who has lost their immunization record might wonder whether they should get a blood test done first to see if they've already been vaccinated. Often, their health care provider will recommend getting the vaccine rather than a blood test because the extra dose of vaccine will boost any existing immunity. Also, blood tests aren't always accurate and, in some cases, may not be available.

WHAT SHOULD I DO IF I MISSED A DOSE OF VACCINE?

Most vaccines are given in multiple doses. Some, like the DTaP vaccine, are given as a series of five shots with the first few doses separated by a couple of months. Others, like the MMR vaccine, are given as a series of two shots, separated by a few years. But if you miss a dose, do you have to start over? No. You can just pick up where you left off. Because your immune system will "remember" the pathogen introduced during previous doses, you don't need to start over.

SHOULD HEALTHY PEOPLE LIVING WITH A PERSON WHO IS IMMUNE-COMPROMISED BE VACCINATED?

Because they are unable to make an adequate immune response, people who are severely immune-compromised—like those receiving long-term steroids for asthma, chemotherapy for cancer, or immune-suppressive therapy for a rheumatologic disease—cannot be vaccinated. But what about those who live with them? The good news is that the only routine vaccine that cannot be given to healthy people living with a person who is immune compromised is the oral polio vaccine (which is a live, weakened vaccine). But, that vaccine has not been used in the United States since 2000. All other live, weakened viral vaccines (chickenpox, influenza [nasal spray], MMR, and rotavirus) can be given. Those who receive these vaccines rarely transmit the vaccine virus to others, but when they do, the vaccine virus is so weak that it doesn't cause harm. People who are immune compromised benefit when those around them are protected against infectious diseases (see "Is It My Social Responsibility to Get Vaccinated?").

DO VACCINES GIVEN TO CHILDREN BEING ADOPTED FROM OTHER COUNTRIES COUNT?

Although in the past, countries outside the United States produced some vaccines that were not adequately potent, today, most vaccines produced worldwide meet quality-control standards. As a rule, vaccines administered outside the United States can be accepted, assuming that administrations are adequately documented and given according to the U.S. schedule, meaning that the minimum ages and the intervals between vaccine doses are the same.

A few general rules:

Chickenpox and pneumococcus. These vaccines are rarely given outside the United States.

MMR. Internationally adopted children sometimes have a vaccine record that states "MMR" even though only the single-component measles vaccine was given. The easiest way to resolve the question of MMR vaccination is to revaccinate with one or two doses of MMR vaccine (see the section titled "Measles, Mumps, and Rubella"). Even if the child has already received MMR vaccine, the extra dose is unlikely to cause a safety problem (see "Is an Extra Dose of Vaccine Harmful?").

Hib. This vaccine is occasionally given outside the United States. Because accurate blood testing in young children is difficult and because adverse events following receipt of Hib vaccine are rare, it is probably best to give the vaccine according to age (see the section titled "*Haemophilus influenzae* type b"): children two to five years old need only one dose of vaccine, and those older than five years don't need to be vaccinated.

Hepatitis A. Children without documented vaccination should get the hepatitis A vaccine if they are more than twelve months old. If vaccination is in question, serological testing can reliably detect whether a child has had this vaccine or been exposed to the disease before coming to the United States.

Hepatitis B. If documentation shows that the child has received at least three doses of hepatitis B vaccine, and if at least one dose was given when the child was more than twenty-four weeks old, the child can be considered protected.

Polio. If a child started the polio series of vaccinations by receiving the oral polio vaccine outside the United States, it is safe for them to receive the polio shot to complete the series in the United States, where only the shot is available. Indeed, most countries that use the oral polio vaccine often give a dose of the polio shot first. This situation is similar to the schedule used in the United States between 1996 and 1998, when infants received two polio shots followed by two doses of the oral polio vaccine.

DTaP. This is probably the toughest set of vaccinations to figure out. If documentation shows that the child has received three or more doses of DTaP or DTP vaccine (see the section titled

"Diphtheria, Tetanus, and Pertussis"), it would be reasonable to do serological testing to see whether the child has antibodies to diphtheria and tetanus toxins (a reliable test to determine pertussis immunity doesn't exist). Alternatively, when three or more doses of DTaP or DTP vaccine are documented, a single booster dose of DTaP can be given, followed by serological testing one month later. In both cases—assuming protective antibodies have been detected—booster doses can be given later according to the U.S. schedule. If serological results are unclear, children should be vaccinated with all recommended doses based on the U.S. schedule.

Because of variations in vaccine products and dosing schedules across countries, each situation is unique. Therefore, it is often useful to get help from your health care provider or local public health officials to determine which vaccines are needed and when.

THINGS TO DO

It's important to remember that measles, hepatitis A, and hepatitis B are common infections worldwide. If not already immunized, people living in the home of an internationally adopted child should receive MMR, hepatitis A, and hepatitis B vaccines, preferably a few weeks or months before the child arrives or before going abroad to get the child. Talk with your health care provider to determine your vaccination needs and an appropriate schedule to ensure immunity before a potential for exposure.

Reference

Centers for Disease Control and Prevention. "General Recommendations on Immunization: Recommendations of the Advisory Committee on Immunization Practices." *Morbidity and Mortality Weekly Report* 55 (2006): 33–35.

WHICH VACCINES SHOULD BE CONSIDERED WHEN TRAVELING INTERNATIONALLY?

When traveling internationally, a travel medicine expert can be extremely helpful. These health care providers specialize in health-related issues associated with international travel, including vaccinations. A person's vaccination needs are often based not only on the destination but also other factors, some of which include the duration of the trip, the type of community (e.g., rural or urban) they will be staying in, and the types of activities they will be doing. As such, a travel medicine expert can offer planning guidance and information about how to protect yourself during and after your trip. You can find a travel medicine clinic or provider from directories offered on the websites of the International Society of Travel Medicine (https://www.istm.org) and the American Society of Tropical Medicine and Hygiene (https://www.astmh .org/for-astmh-members/clinical-consultants-directory).

You can also check out the travel website of the Centers for Disease Control and Prevention (https://wwwnc.cdc.gov/travel), which offers country-specific information, a compilation of current travel warnings, and other resources.

Some required vaccines might be available only at a local travel clinic, and some may require multiple doses. Also, not all insurance policies cover travel vaccines, so you might have to pay for some out of pocket. For these reasons, it is important to give yourself plenty of time to address your vaccination and other health-related needs before traveling.

INDIVIDUAL VACCINES

VACCINES IN THE FIRST YEAR OF LIFE

HEPATITIS B

HEPATITIS B: THE DISEASE

Newborns and sexually transmitted infections aren't typically discussed in the same conversation, so many parents wonder why their baby needs a hepatitis B vaccine before leaving the nursery.

What Is Hepatitis B?

Hepatitis B is a virus that is transmitted most commonly from one person to another by blood. Because as many as one billion infectious viruses can be found in a milliliter (a fifth of a teaspoon) of blood, the amount of blood necessary to transmit the infection is minuscule. Indeed, invisible amounts of blood from an infected person can be found in unusual places, such as toothbrushes, and can be infectious for up to a week.

Before the hepatitis B vaccine was routinely recommended for infants in 1991, about sixteen thousand children less than ten years old were infected with the virus every year. Many of these children got hepatitis B while passing through the birth canal of an infected mother, but some caught it from someone else who was infected. That's why it's so important to be immunized early.

ONE PERSON'S STORY

"We had felt so lucky. Matt, born in Korea, joined our family in 1984. Soon after he came home, he was diagnosed as a hepatitis B carrier. . . . A specialist explained the consequences of hepatitis B, including the risk of liver cancer, the risk of infection for anyone handling the child's body fluids, and the importance of vaccinations for the whole family. . . . We began training our little corner of the world in how anyone should handle someone else's blood, and I dealt with all diapers, spit, etc. We all got our vaccinations. . . . We explained to Matt's teachers that he had inherited a blood disorder and they needed to wear gloves if they had to handle any body fluids. I had a private conversation with the school nurse. No one ever asked questions. I knew of parents who could not find day care or friends for their child with hepatitis B. So, we felt lucky.

As a very little boy, Matt learned that he in particular must not share a toothbrush or razor and must be careful about any blood contact. He learned earlier than most about his liver and that he must always protect it. We talked about the importance of a healthy diet, exercise, and avoiding alcohol."

This family's story took a tragic turn when another of their adopted sons was incorrectly determined not to have hepatitis B. *Source*: Wise, Helen. "One Family's Story: Living with Hepatitis B." Immunize.org. Originally published 12/9/2004. https://www.vaccineinformation.org/testimonies/andrew-wise/

What Are the Symptoms of Hepatitis B?

Hepatitis B infections occur in four forms:

- *Infection with symptoms*: Symptoms include fever, vomiting, nausea, aversion to food, abdominal pain, headache, muscle and joint pain, rash, and dark urine, followed a few days later by jaundice (yellowing of the skin and eyes). Jaundice can last for a few weeks and is often accompanied by discoloration of feces (light or gray color) and an enlargement and tenderness of the liver. Fatigue and general feelings of discomfort usually last for several weeks after other symptoms have resolved. Symptoms first appear one to two months after exposure to hepatitis B virus. About 60 of 100 people in the United States with symptomatic hepatitis B infection will be hospitalized.

- *Infection without symptoms*: This form of disease occurs in most children and about half of adults who are infected. Because there are no symptoms, these people usually aren't aware they've been infected—but they're still contagious.
- *Infection with complications*: This form of disease occurs in about two of 100 people infected with hepatitis B virus. Complications include confusion, jerking movements (particularly of the hands), disorientation, extreme sleepiness, semiconsciousness, and coma: all symptoms of severe liver damage. About 25 of 100 people with severe liver damage will die unless they receive a liver transplant.
- *Long-lasting or chronic infection*: This occurs in about 5 of 100 people infected with hepatitis B virus. Infants and young children are *much* more likely to suffer chronic infections than those who are infected when they are older. Although people with chronic infection are highly contagious, they often don't exhibit any symptoms. People with chronic infection typically develop cirrhosis (severe liver damage), leading to liver failure or liver cancer.

DID YOU KNOW?

People with chronic hepatitis B infection are called carriers. Hepatitis B virus reproduces in carriers for at least six months and often for years. However, because many carriers don't have symptoms, they don't know they're infected and therefore contagious to others. That's why hepatitis B virus is called a silent epidemic. About a million people in the United States are chronic carriers.

DID YOU KNOW?

Globally, hepatitis B virus is the most common cause of fatal liver cancer. About four of every 10 liver cancer deaths are the result of hepatitis B infection. Hepatitis C and alcohol use are the next most common causes of death from liver cancer, responsible for three of 10 and two of 10 cases, respectively.

HEPATITIS B: THE VACCINE
What Is the Hepatitis B Vaccine?

Four hepatitis B vaccines are available.

Infants and children up to eighteen years of age: At the time of writing, two of the four hepatitis B vaccines (Engerix-B and Recombivax HB) can be used in infants and children up to eighteen years of age. Both vaccines use only a single protein from the surface of the virus to generate protective immunity (see "How Are Vaccines Made?"). The protein is produced in yeast cells and purified. As a result, the vaccine contains only the hepatitis B surface protein, a small amount of residual yeast proteins, and aluminum salt as an adjuvant. The aluminum salt is used to enhance the immune response so that less viral protein is needed (see "Do Vaccines Contain Harmful Adjuvants Like Aluminum?").

Adults (eighteen years of age and older): Adults can also receive Engerix-B or Recombivax HB vaccine (in age-appropriate doses); however, because some adults did not gain immunity after receiving one of these vaccines, a few other options have become available. The first, Heplisav-B, is also made using the hepatitis B surface protein produced in yeast cells; however, it contains a different adjuvant called CpG 1018. This adjuvant is composed of a short stretch of two nucleotides, cytosine and guanine. Nucleotides are the building blocks of DNA. CpG 1018 has been shown to be safe and improve the immune response in older people. The second, PreHevbrio, contains three hepatitis B surface proteins produced by mammalian cells in a laboratory setting. PreHevbrio contains aluminum salt as an adjuvant. Because this vaccine is made in mammalian cells, very small amounts of mammalian cell proteins (nanograms [billionths of a gram]) and DNA (picograms [trillionths of a gram]) can be detected in the final vaccine.

Who Should Get the Hepatitis B Vaccine?

The American Academy of Pediatrics (AAP) and the Centers for Disease Control and Prevention (CDC) recommend three doses of the hepatitis B vaccine for all children, to be given at birth, one to two months of age, and between six and eighteen months of age. The first dose is usually given before the newborn leaves the hospital.

Older children and adults up to fifty-nine years of age who were not previously vaccinated against hepatitis B should receive two or three doses, depending on which vaccine they receive.

Previously unvaccinated people sixty years of age and older who have known risk factors should also be vaccinated. Those considered at increased risk include individuals with chronic liver disease, diabetes, or HIV; those who currently or recently used injection drugs; those who are incarcerated; those traveling to countries with a high prevalence of hepatitis B; and those who face increased risk of exposure to hepatitis B–positive blood based on living conditions, occupation, sexual practices, or need for dialysis.

Individuals sixty years of age and older who are unvaccinated but do not have risk factors may also get vaccinated if they so choose.

Does the Hepatitis B Vaccine Work?

After two doses of vaccine, more than half of infants will be protected from hepatitis B; after three doses, at least 98 of 100 full-term infants will be protected. Rates of protection are slightly lower in preterm infants who weigh less than 2,000 grams, so this group is recommended to get their first dose of hepatitis B vaccine when they leave the hospital or one month after birth, whichever occurs first. In the United States, hepatitis B vaccine has virtually eliminated the disease in children.

More than nine of 10 older children and adults younger than forty years of age will be protected after receiving all recommended doses of hepatitis B vaccine. Because the immune system weakens with age, responses to hepatitis B vaccine are more variable after forty years of age (about seven of 10 are protected). The exception to this is when older adults get Heplisav-B, as the adjuvant in that vaccine affords better protection. Studies showed that as many as nine or 10 of every 10 adults are protected after receipt of that version.

DID YOU KNOW?

Hepatitis B vaccine was the first vaccine to prevent a known cause of cancer in people. The human papillomavirus (HPV) vaccine, which prevents the only known cause of cervical cancer, was the second (see the section titled "Human Papillomavirus").

DID YOU KNOW?

Studies have shown that the protection afforded by hepatitis B vaccine lasts for decades. As such, by eliminating hepatitis B in children, we can expect that the main cause of liver cancer will change as they become adults.

Who Should Avoid or Delay Getting Hepatitis B Vaccine?

People who have had a severe allergic reaction to previous doses of hepatitis B vaccine should not get additional doses, and those who are moderately or severely ill should delay getting the vaccine until they are feeling better, particularly to avoid confusion over whether symptoms they experience are from the vaccination or the current illness.

What Are the Side Effects of the Vaccine?

Reactions to hepatitis B vaccine, such as pain at the injection site, mild fever, headache, fatigue, and irritability, have been reported. However, studies have shown that these symptoms do not occur more often in vaccinated individuals than in those injected with a placebo. The vaccine can rarely cause a severe allergic reaction in about one of one million recipients.

Why Get the Hepatitis B Vaccine?

1. *Hepatitis B virus is around.* About 14,000 to 18,000 hepatitis B infections causing about 1,400 to 1,500 deaths occur every year in the United States.

2. *Not everyone with hepatitis B infection knows they're infected.* Almost all children and more than half of adults infected with hepatitis B virus have no symptoms—but they're still contagious. Based on health data, it's estimated that about one million people in the United States are chronically infected and that about 10,000 to 12,000 more become chronically infected every year. However, the number of chronically infected people may actually be twice as high based on comparison of demographic groups with higher rates, census data, and rates of hepatitis B in countries from which migrants come. Regardless of which figure is more accurate, any chronically infected person can transmit hepatitis B to others.

3. *Outcomes tend to be worse in younger people.* Younger people are less likely to have symptoms yet they are more likely to develop a long-term infection, liver damage, and liver cancer. Therefore, protecting children is critical for decreasing their lifetime risk.

4. *The vaccine is safe.* Severe allergic reactions to the vaccine are extraordinarily rare.

HEPATITIS B: OTHER THINGS YOU MIGHT HAVE WONDERED ABOUT

Newborns and Sexually Transmitted Infections

When hepatitis B vaccine first became available in 1981, the AAP and CDC recommended it for high-risk groups, such as health care providers, men who have sex with men, injection drug users, and babies born to infected mothers. Unfortunately, this strategy didn't protect thousands of children under the age of ten who were infected with hepatitis B virus every year from sources other than their mothers, often a family member or family friend who didn't know they were infected. Because children are at higher risk of long-term infection and subsequent liver damage and because those with chronic infections are more likely to transmit the disease, the AAP and CDC recommended in 1991 that all newborns receive the hepatitis B vaccine. Since that time, the disease has been almost completely eliminated in children less than eighteen years of age.

Types of Hepatitis

Hepatitis B is one of several viruses that cause hepatitis. Four other hepatitis viruses can also cause disease: hepatitis A, hepatitis C, hepatitis D, and hepatitis E. These viruses differ in their size, structure, and type of genetic material. In some cases, they also differ in how they're spread. Hepatitis C and D are spread similarly to hepatitis B: through blood and body fluids; hepatitis A and E are spread through feces and contaminated food and water. Because hepatitis B virus is spread primarily through blood, it used to be called serum hepatitis; hepatitis A virus, spread more casually, was once called infectious hepatitis. Hepatitis A and B are the only hepatitis viruses preventable by vaccine.

Extra Dose of Vaccine

Because of combination vaccines, young children sometimes inadvertently get a fourth dose of hepatitis B vaccine. The extra dose does not increase the rate of occurrence of side effects; instead, it boosts the immune response (see "Is an extra dose of vaccine harmful?").

Hepatitis B: Additional Resources

ONLINE INFORMATION

"Hepatitis B": https://media.chop.edu/data/files/pdfs/vec-hepatitis-b-infographic.pdf

"Hepatitis B": https://www.vaccineinformation.org/diseases/hepatitis-b/

"Hepatitis B Vaccine": https://www.voicesforvaccines.org/vaccine-information/hepatitisb/

"Hepatitis B: What You Should Know": https://media.chop.edu/data/files/pdfs/vaccine-education-center-hepatitis-b.pdf

"A Look at Each Vaccine: Hepatitis B Vaccine": https://www.chop.edu/centers-programs/vaccine-education-center/vaccine-details/vaccine-hepatitis-b-vaccine

"Talking About Vaccines with Dr. Paul Offit: News Briefs – May 2018 – New Hepatitis B Vaccine for Adults": https://www.chop.edu/video/talking-about-vaccines-dr-paul-offit-news-briefs-may-2018-new-hepatitis-b-vaccine-adults

"Why Are Adults 19 to 59 Recommended to Get the Hepatitis B Vaccine?":https://www.chop.edu/centers-programs/vaccine-education-center/video/why-are-adults-19-59-recommended-get-hepatitis-b-vaccine

"Why Do Newborns Get the Hepatitis B Vaccine?": https://www.chop.edu/centers-programs/vaccine-education-center/video/why-do-newborns-get-hepatitis-b-vaccine

PHOTOS

"Hepatitis B Photos": https://www.vaccineinformation.org/photos/hepatitis-b/

PERSONAL EXPERIENCES

"Story Gallery": https://www.shotbyshot.org/story-gallery (search "hepatitis B")

"Unprotected People Stories: Hepatitis B": https://www.immunize
.org/clinical/vaccine-confidence/unprotected-people/topic/hepb/

SUPPORT GROUPS

Hepatitis B Foundation: dedicated to finding a cure and improving
the quality of life for families around the world affected by hepatitis B: http://www.hepb.org.

DIPHTHERIA, TETANUS, AND PERTUSSIS (DTaP)

DIPHTHERIA, TETANUS, AND PERTUSSIS: THE DISEASES

Vaccines that protect against diphtheria, tetanus, and pertussis are among the oldest available, although, at least in the case of pertussis, newer ones have been made. Despite being used for many years, these vaccines are still necessary. Diphtheria outbreaks continue to occur throughout the world, pertussis is still common in the United States, and tetanus bacteria will always live in the soil, unaffected by immunization rates.

What Is Diphtheria?

Diphtheria has been virtually eliminated from the United States. However, in the early part of the twentieth century, it was one of the most common killers of young children. The bacteria spread easily from one person to another, primarily by coughing or sneezing. Some people carry the bacteria in their nose and throat without becoming ill, but they can still spread the disease to others. About 10 of 100 people who get diphtheria die from the disease.

ONE PERSON'S STORY

"The Rev. Roland Sawyer wrote of the 1735 epidemic in his history of Kensington [New Hampshire]. . . . 'Seven families lost 27 children, everyone dying who was taken sick . . . we lost . . . near 90 the first 15 months of the plague.' By 1738 so many Kensington children succumbed to diphtheria 'there were few children left to die.'"

Source: Merchant, Dean. "History in Focus: Diphtheria Epidemic." Seacoastonline.com. June 27, 2008. https://www.seacoastonline.com/story/news/local/exeter-news-letter/2008/06/27/history-in-focus-diphtheria-epidemic/52363287007/.

Symptoms of diphtheria aren't caused by the bacterium alone; rather, they're caused by a toxin (poison) produced by the bacterium. A preparation of antibodies that bind to the toxin—preventing it from causing harm—is called an antitoxin.

DID YOU KNOW?

The antitoxin used to treat diphtheria is produced in horses and first became available in the United States in 1891. Today, diphtheria antitoxin is available only from the Centers for Disease Control and Prevention (CDC).

Thanks to high immunization rates, diphtheria has been virtually eliminated from the United States. But a drop in immunization rates can lead to rapid spread of the disease since infections continue to occur in other parts of the world. Between 2011 and the end of 2021, more than one hundred thousand cases occurred globally.

About five to 10 of every 100 people with diphtheria will die from it; however, immunization status and age affect an individual's risk of dying. Most deaths occur in those who are unvaccinated and those younger than five and older than forty years of age.

What Are the Symptoms of Diphtheria?

People with diphtheria experience the following:

- Thick membrane at the back of the throat that can affect the tonsils, voice box, windpipe, or nose by forming a thick, sticky membrane. Attempts to scrape the membrane cause bleeding. As the membrane gets bigger, it can block the airway, causing suffocation. For this reason, diphtheria has been called the "strangling angel of children"

- Infection limited to the lining of the nose, causing a discharge that contains pus and sometimes blood. Nasal infections, which can be mild and resemble the common cold, occur in about two of 100 people with diphtheria
- Infection of the voice box, causing hoarseness and a "barking" cough that occurs in about 25 of 100 people with diphtheria, mostly children less than four years of age
- Infection of the skin at the site of wounds or burns
- Fever, usually mild
- Sore throat
- Swollen glands, particularly in the neck
- Lack of appetite

Complications of diphtheria can include:

- Damage to the heart muscle, causing an abnormal rhythm, heart failure, and death
- Nerve damage, causing paralysis of the eyes, arms, legs, and diaphragm
- Suffocation as a result of the thick membrane at the back of the throat completely obstructing the airway; a tracheostomy (a hole cut into the windpipe) is sometimes necessary to allow breathing

What Is Tetanus?

Tetanus, caused by a bacterium found in the soil, is unique in that it is the only vaccine-preventable disease not transmitted from person to person. Similar to diphtheria, the symptoms of tetanus are caused by a toxin. People get tetanus when the bacteria enter the skin through a wound, such as those from surgery, burns, punctures, ear or dental infections, animal bites, abortions, or pregnancy. Because tetanus can cause muscle spasms of the head and neck, it is commonly known as lockjaw. About 10 of 100 people with tetanus die from the disease. Those most likely to die include people over sixty years of age and those who have not been vaccinated.

What Are the Symptoms of Tetanus?

People with tetanus experience the following:

- Spasms of the jaw and face; this is the most common symptom, occurring in about 90 of 100 infected people
- Spasms of other muscles, including those in the neck, back, abdomen, arms, and legs; spasms tend to develop from the head downward
- Sudden, painful seizure-like spasms that involve most muscles, often triggered by loud noises
- Difficulty swallowing
- Sweating
- Increased blood pressure
- Increased heart rate

ONE PERSON'S STORY

John Roebling Sr., the chief engineer during construction of the Brooklyn Bridge, died from tetanus: "Then the hideous seizures began, set off by the slightest disturbance. His room was kept dark, the long shades drawn against the July sun, and everyone who had reason to go in or out did so as softly as humanly possible. But then a window shade would rattle in the breeze or someone would inadvertently brush against the side of his bed, a door would squeak or there would be a noise from the street below, and he would go into a convulsion, the sight of which was something they would all live with the rest of their lives. All at once his whole body would lift off the bed and double backward with a fierce, awful jerk, his every muscle clenched in violent contraction. Sweat streamed from his body, but he made no sound, not even a groan, because during the spasm his whole chest wall was frozen hard.

"He was being horribly destroyed before their eyes and there was not a thing any of them could do about it. Moreover, as nearly always happens with lockjaw, his mind remained as clear as ever, and this made the sight of his suffering all the more unbearable. They all knew the terrible, titanic battle going on behind those blazing eyes and the ghastly smile that stayed fixed like concrete on his ashen face throughout everything that was happening to him. When the seizures passed, he generally slipped into a coma. But even toward the end, there were hours when he would lie there perfectly still in the darkened room staring straight up at the ceiling, one of his family sitting motionless beside him. During the final few days there were tears streaking down his face."

From *The Great Bridge* by David McCullough, copyright © 1972, 2001 by David McCullough. Reprinted with the permission of Simon & Schuster, Inc. All rights reserved.

Complications of tetanus can include:

- Difficulty breathing caused by spasms of the vocal cords and muscles used for breathing
- Fractures of the spine and other bones caused by continued severe spasms
- Pneumonia caused by acids or bacteria in the mouth that enter the windpipe and travel to the lungs during a spasm

What Is Pertussis?

Pertussis, or whooping cough, is known by the sound that infected children make while trying to cough up the thick, sticky mucus that covers the back of their throats. The characteristic whoop, caused by breathing in against a narrowed windpipe, is a sound that parents never forget. (To hear what a pertussis cough sounds like, visit https://www.youtube.com/watch?v=DB7oizafC1Y.) The bacteria that cause pertussis are easily spread from one person to another by coughing or sneezing; indeed, if ten susceptible people are in a room with an infected person, eight are likely to also develop pertussis. About 20 of 100 people with pertussis will be hospitalized, and about one of five hundred will die from the disease.

ONE PERSON'S STORY

This story, from Dr. Marina Catallozzi, describes a family she saw during her pediatric residency at the Children's Hospital of Philadelphia. She recalls, "Her [a mother's] two-month-old came in, wasn't breathing for a time, needed a breathing tube, was in the intensive care nursery. The two-year-old was coughing and vomiting, unable to eat for a week. The four-year-old was coughing so horribly that she would ask for help before going into her coughing spasms. There was a seven-year-old and a seventeen-year-old, and each of those children missed school for several weeks. The whole family was adversely affected from something that could have been prevented. It's really hard as a caretaker to see the effect of choosing not to immunize."

Source: "Vaccines: Separating Fact from Fear." Vaccine Education Center at the Children's Hospital of Philadelphia. Last reviewed July 23, 2014. https://www.chop.edu/centers-programs/vaccine-education-center /video/vaccines-separating-fact-fear.

DID YOU KNOW?

Many infectious diseases are transmitted from young children to teenagers and adults. But not pertussis. Because immunity doesn't last throughout life, adolescents and adults often get pertussis and transmit it to infants.

What Are the Symptoms of Pertussis?

Unlike diphtheria and tetanus, each of which makes a single toxin, pertussis makes several toxins. These toxins interfere with the lining of the windpipe and lungs, causing intense inflammation. The disease occurs in three stages:

- STAGE 1: Lasts up to two weeks; symptoms are similar to those of a common cold and include runny nose, sneezing, mild fever, and coughing
- STAGE 2: Lasts from one to eight weeks; symptoms include a distinctive cough that occurs in bursts, ending with a long intake of air against a windpipe narrowed by inflammation. Coughing episodes often cause vomiting and exhaustion. Because of the lack of oxygen while coughing, a young child's lips might turn blue. An infected child will have about fifteen coughing spells a day; however, between spells, the child often will not appear to be ill. The coughing spells can also cause difficulty sleeping, nosebleeds, brain hemorrhage, hernias, and broken ribs
- STAGE 3: Lasts for weeks to months, during which time a decrease in the frequency and intensity of coughing spells occurs

DID YOU KNOW?

While most adults with pertussis experience a mild coughing illness, about one in five are more severely affected. Those with more severe disease experience cough for about eight weeks, with about six weeks classified as "violent coughing" that can result in whooping, vomiting, or apnea (temporary stoppage breathing). For many, coughing worsens at night, interfering with sleep.

Complications of pertussis can include:

- Pneumonia, which occurs in about five of 100 people, is the most common cause of death from pertussis
- Seizures

- Swelling of the brain and spinal cord
- Ear infections
- Lack of appetite
- Weight loss
- Urinary incontinence
- Fractured ribs
- Dehydration

DIPHTHERIA, TETANUS, AND PERTUSSIS: THE VACCINES
What Are the Diphtheria, Tetanus, and Pertussis Vaccines?

Vaccines for diphtheria and tetanus are made using similar methods. In each case, the bacteria are grown in a nutrient liquid where they produce the toxins that cause disease. The bacteria are removed by filtration, leaving the toxins, which are then treated with the chemical formaldehyde (see "Do Vaccines Contain Harmful Chemicals Like Formaldehyde?") to inactivate them so they can no longer cause harm. Inactivated toxins are called toxoids. The toxoids are then dried onto an aluminum salt that serves as an adjuvant (see "Do Vaccines Contain Harmful Adjuvants Like Aluminum?"). An adjuvant is used to generate a stronger immune response with lesser quantities of toxoid.

The pertussis vaccine is made by growing bacteria in nutrient broth purifying the toxins and proteins that cause disease and then inactivating them with a chemical like formaldehyde. The original pertussis vaccine, referred to as the whole-cell pertussis vaccine, was made by killing the entire bacterium, which contains about three thousand pertussis proteins. However, as scientists better understood which components of pertussis bacteria caused disease, bacterial toxins and individual proteins were purified away from the bacteria, so the vaccine now contains only two to five pertussis proteins. This newer version is known as the acellular pertussis vaccine (the word *cell* refers to the bacterial cell, which is removed in the newer version).

Vaccines have been available for diphtheria, tetanus, and pertussis since the early 1900s and were first combined into a single shot, called DTP, in 1948. Since then, the vaccines for these three diseases have been variously combined, leading to an alphabet soup of vaccine names:

DTP: contains the diphtheria, tetanus, and whole-cell pertussis vaccines; it was the first combination vaccine for infants and is no longer available in the United States, having been replaced by the DTaP vaccine

DTaP: contains the diphtheria, tetanus, and acellular pertussis vaccines; this vaccine is now used for infants in the United States

DT: contains the diphtheria and tetanus vaccines; this vaccine was used only for children who could not get the pertussis vaccine. It was discontinued in the United States in 2023. However, because some children are unable to get the pertussis vaccine, public health officials are working to develop recommendations with alternative options

Tdap: contains the tetanus, diphtheria, and acellular pertussis vaccines and is used in adolescents and adults. It contains lesser quantities of the diphtheria and pertussis components (hence the lowercase *d* and *p* in the name) than the DTaP vaccine because adolescents and adults who received diphtheria and pertussis vaccinations as children will have some immunity; therefore, a smaller dose is sufficient to boost the immune response

Td: contains only the tetanus and diphtheria vaccines and is used in those aged seven years and older. The quantity of diphtheria vaccine is about one-third to one-quarter that contained in the previous version (DT vaccine) used for young children

Who Should Get the Diphtheria, Tetanus, and Pertussis Vaccines?

The DTaP vaccine is recommended for all children as a series of five shots given at two months, four months, six months, between fifteen and eighteen months, and between four and six years of age. The first three doses are necessary to protect most children, while the fourth dose boosts the immune response and the fifth provides an additional booster before starting school.

Older children are recommended to get one dose of Tdap between eleven and twelve years of age, followed by one dose of either Tdap or Td every ten years thereafter. Teens and adults who have not gotten an adolescent dose of Tdap should get a single dose, followed by the same ten-year pattern of boosters.

A dose of Tdap should also be administered on two other occasions:

- During *every* pregnancy, preferably between twenty-seven and thirty-six weeks of gestation. This is to provide the baby with protection via maternal antibodies in the first few months after birth before they develop antibodies following their own vaccinations (DTaP at two, four, and six months of age)
- Following a wound that requires tetanus vaccination depending on the wound type and time since receipt of the last tetanus-containing vaccine

Who Should Avoid or Delay Getting Diphtheria, Tetanus, and Pertussis Vaccines?

Anyone who has had a severe allergic reaction to a previous dose of DTaP, DT, Tdap, or Td vaccine should not get additional doses. If a person experiences unexplained symptoms related to swelling of the brain (e.g., coma, decreased consciousness, or prolonged seizures) within seven days of getting DTaP or Tdap vaccine, they should not get additional doses of pertussis-containing vaccines. However, they may still be able to get the Td vaccine if they are old enough to receive it.

Some infants who get the DTaP vaccine experience reactions attributable to the pertussis component, including fever of 105°F or higher, shock-like state (called hypotonic-hyporesponsive syndrome), inconsolable crying lasting longer than three hours, or seizures with fever. These infants used to be offered DT for additional doses; however, an option without the pertussis vaccine is currently not available for those younger than seven years of age. Even when DT was available, these infants were not protected from pertussis, so any infant who does not get additional doses of DTaP because of these side effects may still be recommended to get a dose if a pertussis outbreak occurs in their area.

If a person is diagnosed with Guillain-Barré syndrome (GBS) within six weeks of getting a dose of tetanus-containing vaccine, they should speak with their health care provider about whether and when to get additional doses. Similarly, if a person has a reaction that involves severe swelling, pain, redness, and tissue hardening near the injection site (known as an Arthus reaction), they are often advised to wait ten years before getting another dose of tetanus-containing vaccine. However, since tetanus can be fatal and vaccination after exposure can be protective, individuals should discuss their options with a health care provider. Anyone with a worsening neurologic disorder or uncontrolled epilepsy should wait until their condition has stabilized before getting any of these vaccines. Those who are moderately or severely ill should delay vaccination until they are feeling better.

What Are the Side Effects of the Vaccines?

DTaP vaccine is safe but can cause some side effects:

- Pain, redness, or swelling at the injection site occurs in about 30 of 100 vaccine recipients, more frequently in children after the fourth or fifth dose. Swelling can involve the entire arm or leg; however, this reaction does not cause permanent harm, and further doses can still be given.
- Fever of 101°F or higher occurs in about four of 100 infants.
- Drowsiness or crankiness.
- More severe reactions, including fever of 105°F or higher, fever-associated seizures, inconsolable crying for three hours or more, hypotonic-hyporesponsive syndrome; severe reactions occur in about one of ten thousand children and are attributed to the pertussis component.

Tdap and Td vaccines cause a few minor side effects at similar rates:

- Pain, redness, or swelling at the injection site occurs in about 50 of 100 people
- Fever of 100.4°F or higher occurs in about one of 100 people
- General symptoms such as headache, fatigue, or upset stomach

Why Get the Diphtheria, Tetanus, and Pertussis Vaccines?

1. *Pertussis is still around.* Pertussis is often underreported because many adults don't see a doctor for illnesses resulting in a prolonged cough, and older children and adults often spread this infection to young infants for whom it can be life threatening. Between 2000 and 2019, about one in three cases in children younger than one year of age occurred in infants younger than two months of age, a period when they cannot yet get vaccinated. The recommendation for pregnant people to get a dose of Tdap late in pregnancy has helped increase protection for these young infants, but not all pregnant people get vaccinated before delivery.

2. *While most people recover from pertussis, prevention is always the better choice.* Pertussis can be severe. Some people suffer complications such as broken ribs, seizures, and hernias. Others die, particularly infants, who are less capable of clearing mucus from their windpipes than teenagers and adults.

3. *Diphtheria can readily reemerge in the United States.* Between 2011 and 2021, more than one hundred thousand cases of diphtheria occurred globally, and diphtheria isn't a trivial infection; it can cause heart disease, paralysis, airway obstruction, and death.

4. *Tetanus will never go away.* The bacteria that cause tetanus live in the soil and often contaminate wounds, burns, or other breaks in the skin. Because tetanus isn't spread from one person to another, people aren't protected from tetanus by herd immunity (also referred to as community immunity, herd immunity occurs when enough people are immunized so that bacteria or viruses cannot spread, even to those who aren't immunized). Even if

everyone in the world were immunized against tetanus, the risk to an unimmunized person would be the same. Tetanus causes muscle spasms that interfere with breathing and swallowing and can result in bone fractures or even death.

5. *The vaccines are safe.* Although there are some mild side effects and rarely more severe side effects, the benefits of the vaccines clearly outweigh their risks.

DIPHTHERIA, TETANUS, AND PERTUSSIS: OTHER THINGS YOU MIGHT HAVE WONDERED ABOUT

Safety Concerns About the Pertussis Vaccine

No vaccine has generated more questions about safety than the pertussis vaccine, particularly in the early 1980s. On April 19, 1982, a local NBC affiliate in Washington, DC, aired a documentary titled *DPT: Vaccine Roulette.* The program claimed that the pertussis vaccine caused cognitive developmental delay and epilepsy. At the time, the pertussis vaccine was different from the one used today. Called the whole-cell pertussis vaccine, it was made using the whole bacterium. The vaccine was a common cause of pain, redness, and tenderness at the site of injection; fever, including high fever; drowsiness; fretfulness; decreased appetite; prolonged or high-pitched crying; seizures with fever; and hypotonic-hyporesponsive syndrome. In short, the old whole-cell pertussis vaccine had a high rate of side effects. The question was whether the vaccine could also cause permanent brain damage.

In the decade after *DPT: Vaccine Roulette* first aired, researchers examined thousands of children who did or did not receive the whole-cell pertussis vaccine to see whether it caused permanent brain damage, and they found that it didn't. Another ten years passed before researchers developed the genetic tools necessary to determine what was wrong with the children featured on the program. They found that most of the children had probably been born with something called "neuronal sodium channel transport defect," known as Dravet syndrome. This defect causes brain cells to be unusually excitable, resulting in seizures and cognitive developmental delay regardless of whether they received vaccines.

Although the whole-cell pertussis vaccine didn't cause permanent brain damage, many parents (and doctors) who watched the program—or were influenced by the intense media coverage that followed—believed that it had. Today, with the use of the acellular pertussis vaccine—a purer, safer product—the incidence of side effects following vaccination has been dramatically reduced. Unfortunately, for some, however, the fear of the pertussis vaccine has remained.

Protecting Young Infants from Pertussis
Before They Are Fully Vaccinated

Young infants are particularly vulnerable to pertussis because of their small windpipes. Although the first dose of pertussis vaccine is given at two months of age, most infants aren't fully protected until after the third dose at six months. Indeed, of the approximately twenty babies who die every year from pertussis in the United States, most are less than three months old. To protect them, public health officials suggest that pregnant people get vaccinated between twenty-seven and thirty-six weeks of gestation. As the pregnant person's immune system responds to the vaccine, antibodies circulate to the unborn baby, protecting them in the high-risk weeks after birth before they can get their own vaccinations.

Previous recommendations for those who will be around newborns to get a dose of Tdap vaccine before the baby is born, known as cocooning, were not as effective as hoped. However, anyone with symptoms of a respiratory infection should limit their time with the baby as much as possible, and everyone around the baby should maintain good hygiene practices, like washing their hands before touching the baby, refraining from kissing or touching the baby's face, and covering any coughs.

THINGS TO DO

Young infants should be kept away from anyone who is coughing or has cold-like symptoms. People with cold-like symptoms may be in the early stage of pertussis infection, so keeping babies away from them is another way to lessen the chance of infection.

Diphtheria, Tetanus, and Pertussis: Additional Resources

ONLINE INFORMATION

"DTaP (Diphtheria, Tetanus, Pertussis) Vaccine": https://www.voices forvaccines.org/vaccine-information/dtap/

"Which Adults Need a Tdap Vaccine?": https://www.chop.edu/centers -programs/vaccine-education-center/video/which-adults-need -tdap-vaccine

"Diphtheria": https://www.vaccineinformation.org/diseases/diphtheria/

"A Look at Each Vaccine: Diphtheria, Tetanus and Pertussis Vaccines": https://www.chop.edu/centers-programs/vaccine-education -center/vaccine-details/diphtheria-tetanus-and-pertussis-vaccines

"Tetanus (Lockjaw)": https://www.vaccineinformation.org/diseases /tetanus/

"Tetanus: What You Should Know": https://media.chop.edu/data/files /pdfs/vaccine-education-center-tetanus-qa-special-topics.pdf

"Doctors Talk: Pertussis": https://www.chop.edu/centers-programs /vaccine-education-center/video/doctors-talk-pertussis

"Pertussis: What You Should Know": https://media.chop.edu/data/files /pdfs/vaccine-education-center-pertussis-vaccine.pdf

"What Is That Sound? Whooping Cough": https://www.youtube.com /watch?v=DB7oizafC1Y

"Whooping Cough (Pertussis)": https://www.vaccineinformation.org /diseases/whooping-cough/

PHOTOS

"Diphtheria Photos": https://www.vaccineinformation.org/photos /diphtheria/

"Tetanus Photos": https://www.vaccineinformation.org/photos/tetanus/

"Whooping Cough (Pertussis) Photos": https://www.vaccineinformation
   .org/photos/whooping-cough/

PERSONAL EXPERIENCES

"Story Gallery": https://www.shotbyshot.org/story-gallery/ (search
   "pertussis")

"Unprotected People Stories: Diphtheria": https://www.immunize.org
   /clinical/vaccine-confidence/unprotected-people/topic/diphtheria/

"Unprotected People Stories: Tetanus": https://www.immunize.org
   /clinical/vaccine-confidence/unprotected-people/topic/tetanus/

"Unprotected People Stories: Pertussis": https://www.immunize.org
   /clinical/vaccine-confidence/unprotected-people/topic/pertussis/

PNEUMOCOCCUS

PNEUMOCOCCUS: THE DISEASE

Ear infections. Pneumonia. Meningitis. Bloodstream infections. Sepsis. Death. These can be the outcomes of pneumococcal infections. Pneumococcus is a bacterium that most often takes the severest toll on the youngest and oldest among us. But, it also seizes opportunities to infect the rest of us during short periods of weakened immunity, such as following a viral infection or when one's respiratory tract or immune system is weakened for a more prolonged period, such as can happen from smoking, alcoholism, or a chronic medical condition.

What Is Pneumococcus?

Pneumococcus is a bacterium that often lives harmlessly on the lining of the nose and throat. It is spread from one person to another by coughing, sneezing, and talking. More than ninety types of pneumococcus cause disease. However, only a small number of these are responsible for most disease. For example, thirteen types are responsible for about 75 to 90 percent of cases of severe pneumococcal disease in children less than five years of age depending on which part of the world the child resides. In the United States, these types account for closer to 90 percent of cases.

DID YOU KNOW?

People can carry pneumococcal bacteria in their noses and throats. Although they may not be sick, they can still transmit the bacteria to others. Pneumococcal vaccines have decreased the number of people carrying the bacteria. It's estimated that about one in five children and about one in 10 adults in the United States have pneumococcal bacteria in their noses and throats.

Pneumococcus is an opportunist, often complicating viral infections of the respiratory tract, like influenza and respiratory syncytial virus (RSV). For example, during the 2009–2010 novel H1N1 influenza (swine flu) pandemic, people vaccinated against pneumococcus were less likely to be hospitalized than those who were not.

Although pneumococcal infections can occur at any time of year, they often accompany other respiratory infections so they are more common during the winter and early spring.

What Are the Symptoms of Pneumococcus?

Pneumococcus causes several illnesses:

- *Pneumonia:* This occurs most commonly in adults. Symptoms include fever, chills, chest pain, cough, shortness of breath, rapid breathing, increased heart rate, weakness, and, in some cases, nausea, vomiting, and headache. Occasionally, complications such as pericarditis (inflammation of the outer lining of the heart) or lung abscesses can occur. About five of 100 people with pneumococcal pneumonia die from the disease.
- *Sepsis:* This occurs most commonly in older people and very young infants; about 20 of 100 people with sepsis die from the infection.
- *Meningitis:* People with pneumococcal meningitis have symptoms similar to those of other bacterial causes of meningitis (e.g., meningococcus, *Haemophilus influenzae* type b [Hib]), including headache, tiredness, vomiting, irritability, fever, stiff neck, seizures, and coma. About 30 of 100 people with meningitis die from the disease.
- *Ear infections:* Millions of ear infections occur in children in the United States every year; pneumococcus is one of the three most common bacterial causes of ear infections in children.

ONE PERSON'S STORY

"My husband was admitted [to the hospital] on Tuesday evening. On Wednesday, his skin appeared to be burned and the muscles in his arms and legs started to blister. The doctors explained that my husband was septic from the bacteria which had invaded his blood system. After the blisters, my husband's hands and feet started to lose circulation. His hands started to turn black, and his feet began to look dried up. He was on dialysis every day; his liver failed, and he could not breathe on his own. Eventually his bowels stopped functioning. My husband was a really nice guy who deserved to have the knowledge needed to save his life; however, it was not provided to us. . . . As a result of not getting the vaccine against this deadly bacterium, my husband died on August 5, 2007. I continue to be devastated by my loss; it is all so unbelievable to me."

Source: Sands-Duff, Martha. "Parents PACK Personal Stories – Pneumococcus: Pneumococcal Vaccine for People Without a Healthy Spleen." Vaccine Education Center at the Children's Hospital of Philadelphia. Last reviewed May 26, 2020. https://www.chop.edu/centers -programs/parents-pack/personal-stories/pneumococcus.

DID YOU KNOW?

Ear infections account for about twenty million visits to pediatricians' offices every year, making them one of the most common reasons for childhood sick visits.

PNEUMOCOCCUS: THE VACCINE

What Is the Pneumococcal Vaccine?

Three pneumococcal vaccines are currently available in the United States. One (known as PPSV23) is composed of the complex sugar coating (polysaccharide) from twenty-three types of pneumococcus. This version is most often used only in older adults and high-risk individuals because people don't always make a good immune response to the polysaccharides in this vaccine. The other two vaccines (known as PCV15 and PCV20) are made by attaching the polysaccharide from fifteen or twenty types of pneumococcus to a "helper" protein that allows recipients to make a better immune response than they do to the polysaccharide alone. Vaccines made by linking bacterial polysaccharides to helper proteins are called conjugate vaccines; the meningococcal and Hib vaccines are made in a manner identical to the conjugate pneumococcal vaccine.

DID YOU KNOW?

The first conjugate pneumococcal vaccine, available in 2000, protected against seven types of pneumococcus. It was called PCV7. In 2010, PCV7 was replaced with PCV13, which, as the name suggests, protected against thirteen types of pneumococcal bacteria. In June 2023, the Advisory Committee on Immunization Practices, a group of experts who advise the CDC, recommended using only PCV15 or PCV20 in infants and high-risk individuals. As such, it is likely that PCV13 will also fade into vaccine history books.

Does the Pneumococcal Vaccine Work?

The fifteen to twenty different polysaccharides contained in the conjugate pneumococcal vaccine prevent about 90 of 100 bloodstream infections, about 90 percent of 100 cases of meningitis, and about 70 of 100 ear infections caused by pneumococcus in children younger than six years of age.

Adults have benefited from pneumococcal vaccination of children; however, each year, many high-risk and older adults are still hospitalized with more severe complications of pneumococcal infection, like pneumonia, bloodstream infections, and meningitis. The vaccines approved for use in adults (PPSV23, PCV15, and PCV20) are estimated to prevent 70 to 80 of 100 cases caused by these complications.

DID YOU KNOW?

Pneumococcal vaccination of children has also led to a decline in pneumococcal infections in elderly adults. This phenomenon is known as herd immunity (see "Is It My Social Responsibility to Get Vaccinated?" and "Is Herd Immunity Real?").

Who Should Get the Pneumococcal Vaccine?

The pneumococcal vaccine is recommended for all infants at two, four, and six months of age and between twelve and fifteen months of age. Infants can receive either the PCV15 or PCV20 vaccine for these four doses.

Adults sixty-five years of age and older are also recommended to get pneumococcal vaccine. The number of doses, timing, and which type depends on their pneumococcal vaccination history. The vaccines that may be recommended include PCV15, PCV20, and PPSV23. Adults should speak to their health care provider, pharmacist, or local public health officials for help determining their individual pneumococcal vaccine needs.

Those two to sixty-four years of age at high risk for pneumococcus should also receive pneumococcal vaccine if they have not previously. High-risk groups include those with cochlear implants; sickle cell disease; some blood-based or malignant conditions, including Hodgkin disease, leukemia, lymphoma, and multiple myeloma; HIV; alcoholism; cerebrospinal fluid (CSF) leak; certain immune-compromising conditions such as chronic heart, lung, liver, or kidney disease; and diabetes; as well as those who have received a solid organ transplant and those without a spleen. Cigarette smokers are also considered high risk and should be vaccinated.

Who Should Delay or Avoid Getting the Pneumococcal Vaccine?

People who are moderately or severely ill should delay getting the pneumococcal vaccine, and anyone who has had a severe allergic reaction to previous doses should not get additional doses. Those who have had a severe allergic reaction to any diphtheria-containing vaccine should not receive pneumococcal conjugate vaccines (PCV15 or PCV20) due to the use of a type of diphtheria toxin as the helper protein.

What Are the Side Effects of the Pneumococcal Vaccine?

The pneumococcal conjugate vaccine is safe; however, it can cause some mild side effects, including:

- Pain or redness at the injection site occurs for up to two days in five to 50 of 100 recipients. In some cases, the reaction is severe enough that it hurts to move the arm or leg that was injected; these reactions are most common after the fourth dose in infants.
- Fever higher than 102°F one or two days after vaccination in about 10 of 100 people.
- Decreased appetite and irritability are common in babies.

Why Get the Pneumococcal Vaccine?

1. *Pneumococcal infections are common.* Pneumococcus causes pneumonia, bloodstream infection, and meningitis every year in the United States. And because the bacteria often live silently on the lining of the nose and throat in some healthy people, you don't know who is contagious.
2. *Some types of pneumococcus no longer respond readily to antibiotics.* Although bacterial resistance to antibiotics has started to decline, it hasn't gone away.
3. *Pneumococcal infections often complicate other infections.* Pneumococcus can complicate other respiratory infections, such as influenza, causing severe and occasionally fatal disease, particularly in older adults and those in high-risk groups.
4. *The pneumococcal vaccine works.* Studies have shown that people with severe pneumococcal disease were less likely to have gotten the vaccine or were infected with a type of pneumococcus not

contained in an older, seven-component version of the vaccine. Fortunately, now that the fifteen- and twenty-component vaccines are available, the number of infections caused by types of pneumococcus not contained in the vaccine should decrease even more.

5. *The vaccine is safe.* Side effects are minor and uncommon.

PNEUMOCOCCUS: OTHER THINGS YOU MIGHT HAVE WONDERED ABOUT

Causes of Meningitis

Meningitis—an infection of the lining of the brain and spinal cord—can be caused by viruses or bacteria. Bacterial meningitis tends to be more severe and is often life threatening. Not all cases of bacterial meningitis can be prevented by vaccination:

- Some types of pneumococcus are not contained in the vaccine.
- Bacteria other than pneumococcus can cause meningitis. Some of these are also preventable by vaccines, including *Haemophilus influenzae* type b (Hib) and meningococcus, but others, such as *Listeria monocytogenes* and group B *Streptococcus*, aren't.
- Vaccine-preventable viruses that cause meningitis include mumps and polio, but vaccines aren't available for other viruses that cause meningitis, such as enteroviruses.

> **DID YOU KNOW?**
>
> Since the introduction of the Hib vaccine, pneumococcus has become the most common cause of bacterial meningitis in children less than five years of age. It is also the most common cause of bacterial meningitis in adults.

Antibiotics

In the 1940s, antibiotics such as penicillin were discovered to effectively treat pneumococcal infections, so interest in developing a vaccine declined. By the 1960s, two findings led researchers back to working on a vaccine:

- Despite treatment with antibiotics, some people still died from pneumococcal disease; antibiotics were not always effective in cases of rapid and overwhelming bloodstream infection and meningitis.
- Pneumococcal bacteria evolved so that some were no longer easily treatable with antibiotics. Fortunately, since the introduction of conjugate pneumococcal vaccines, this trend has started to reverse; however, it is unlikely to go away.

Additional Resources

ONLINE INFORMATION

"A Look at Each Vaccine: Pneumococcal Vaccine": https://www.chop.edu/centers-programs/vaccine-education-center/vaccine-details/pneumococcal-vaccine

"Pneumococcal Disease": https://www.vaccineinformation.org/diseases/pneumococcal/

"Pneumococcus: What You Should Know": https://media.chop.edu/data/files/pdfs/vaccine-education-center-pneumococcus.pdf

PHOTOS

"Pneumococcal Photos": https://www.vaccineinformation.org/photos/pneumococcal/

PERSONAL EXPERIENCES

"Parents PACK Personal Stories – Pneumococcus": https://www.chop.edu/centers-programs/parents-pack/personal-stories/pneumococcus

"Story Gallery": https://www.shotbyshot.org/story-gallery/ (search "pneumococcal")

"Unprotected People Stories: Pneumococcal": https://www.immunize.org/clinical/vaccine-confidence/unprotected-people/topic/pneumococcal/

ROTAVIRUS

ROTAVIRUS: THE DISEASE

Sudden high fever, vomiting, and diarrhea that lasts up to a week—if you have older children, you probably remember this illness. And if it happened in the winter and your child was less than three years old, the most likely cause was rotavirus. Before the vaccine was first used in the United States in 2006, all children were infected with rotavirus by five years of age. Indeed, rotavirus infects children throughout the world, independent of the level of sanitation in the country or hygiene in the home. About 20 of 100 unvaccinated children with a first-time rotavirus infection need medical care for dehydration (water loss).

What Is Rotavirus?

Rotavirus infects the young of virtually all mammalian and some avian species. Typically, species barriers are high, meaning that cow rotaviruses cause disease in calves, and human rotaviruses cause disease in babies, but not vice versa. Rotavirus is transmitted from infected people in their feces, typically from poorly washed hands, toys, or contaminated surfaces.

> **THINGS TO DO**
>
> Rotaviruses can be killed with rubbing alcohol, bleach, or disinfectant solutions. Toys that children put into their mouths can be washed with soap and water and then disinfected. In childcare settings, this should be done daily.

Rotavirus infections spread throughout the United States every year, beginning in November or December in the Southwest and moving to the Northeast by April or May. In tropical climates, the disease occurs during cooler, drier months.

WHAT ARE THE SYMPTOMS OF ROTAVIRUS?

Although some infants with rotavirus do not have symptoms, most experience the following:

- Fever higher than 102°F occurs in about 33 of 100 infected infants
- Watery diarrhea
- Vomiting

Symptoms last from three days to a week and are most severe during the first rotavirus infection. In severe cases, vomiting and diarrhea can lead to dehydration, sodium imbalance, and hospitalization. Children who are immune compromised may develop a longer-lasting infection and prolonged diarrhea.

ONE PERSON'S STORY

"The next day, however, our beautiful daughter was once again on the couch unable and unwilling to move. She had been vomiting and suffering from diarrhea for three days. This time we went straight to the emergency room. She was dehydrated and would once again need IV fluids. They attempted to start an IV line in her left arm but ended up blowing all three viable veins. They then tried her right arm, her hands, her feet and even her forehead, but all twelve attempts failed. She was so dehydrated that starting an IV was next to impossible."

Source: Matthys, Brooke. "Parents PACK Personal Stories—Rotavirus: Two Children Hospitalized with Rotavirus." Vaccine Education Center at Children's Hospital of Philadelphia. Last reviewed May 27, 2020. http://www.chop.edu/service/parents-possessing-accessing -communicating-knowledge-about-vaccines/sharing-personal-stories /rotavirus.html.

ROTAVIRUS: THE VACCINE
What Is the Rotavirus Vaccine?

Two rotavirus vaccines are available in the United States. Both are made from live, weakened rotaviruses, and both are given by mouth. The rotavirus vaccine is currently the only routinely recommended childhood vaccine given by mouth in the United States. Previously, the polio vaccine was also administered by mouth (called OPV), but because that vaccine could on rare occasions cause paralysis, the inactivated polio vaccine (called IPV) is now routinely used.

One of the two rotavirus vaccines available in the United States, RotaTeq, became available in 2006. It contains five rotavirus strains. Each strain in the RotaTeq vaccine contains a calf rotavirus that has been altered to include a single protein from a human rotavirus that is important for immunologic protection; these altered viruses are known as reassortant viruses. The cow rotavirus was chosen because it doesn't cause disease in children. The human rotavirus proteins in the five vaccine viruses in RotaTeq were chosen based on which rotaviruses most commonly infect infants.

Another rotavirus vaccine, Rotarix, became available in the United States in 2008. Rotarix contains one human strain of rotavirus that has been weakened in the laboratory so that it can't cause the disease (see "How Are Vaccines Made?").

The two vaccines also differ in that RotaTeq requires three doses and Rotarix requires two doses.

Who Should Get the Rotavirus Vaccine?

The AAP and the CDC recommend rotavirus vaccine for all infants. The vaccine is given by mouth at two months and four months of age; for infants who receive RotaTeq, a third dose is given at six months. The first dose should be given before fifteen weeks of age, and the last dose should not be given after eight months of age. These limitations on vaccine timing are related to the age at which the risk for intussusception, a condition in which the small intestine telescopes into itself causing a blockage, increases during infancy, given the history of rotavirus vaccine and intussusception (see "What Are the Side Effects of the Rotavirus Vaccine?").

Infants who spit out a dose of the rotavirus vaccine don't need to repeat the dose.

Does the Rotavirus Vaccine Work?

Both rotavirus vaccines protect more than 90 of 100 infants from getting moderate to severe rotavirus disease. This means that although vaccinated infants may still be infected with rotavirus, symptoms will be absent or mild.

Who Shouldn't Get the Rotavirus Vaccine?

Infants who have had a severe allergic reaction to a previous dose of rotavirus vaccine or one of its ingredients, those with a previous episode of intussusception, and those diagnosed with a genetic condition characterized as severe combined immunodeficiency (SCID) should not get the rotavirus vaccine. Those with moderate or severe intestinal viral infections should delay getting the vaccine until they have recovered.

What Are the Side Effects of the Rotavirus Vaccine?

Rotavirus vaccines are safe. Vaccination typically doesn't result in many side effects, but babies may be irritable, develop a fever, or experience a small amount of vomiting and diarrhea for a few days afterward.

One rare condition requires specific mention. Intussusception, an intestinal blockage, has been associated with rotavirus infections, and a previous rotavirus vaccine, RotaShield, was also associated with a small number of cases, causing it to be removed from use in the United States (see "What Systems Are in Place to Ensure That Vaccines Are Safe?"). Current rotavirus vaccines have also been associated with rare episodes of intussusception; however, when compared with the number of cases caused by rotavirus infection, or even the RotaShield vaccine, the rates have been much lower and not always identifiable in studies trying to assess the risk. Based on existing data and years of experience with this vaccine, the CDC estimates that the rotavirus vaccine results in fifty to sixty additional cases of intussusception each year while preventing fifty thousand hospitalizations and fifty to sixty deaths in the same period.

To reduce the potential for harm caused by intussusception, three safety mechanisms are in place. First, rotavirus vaccination should be completed before eight months of age, a time at which a baby's risk for this condition increases naturally. Second, babies who have had an episode of intussusception should not get the vaccine since previous events increase the risk of future episodes. Third, parents should monitor babies for signs of intussusception in the seven days after vaccination. Symptoms of intussusception include stomach pain and severe crying spells that come and go several times an hour. The baby may pull their legs up to their chest in pain, vomit, or have blood in their feces. If a baby has any of these symptoms, they should be seen by a doctor or taken to the emergency department because intussusception can be a medical emergency if left untreated. While this condition can be scary, parents should be reassured by the fact that tens of millions of doses of both rotavirus vaccines have now been given without consequence. It should be noted that rotavirus disease is also a rare cause of intussusception.

Why Get the Rotavirus Vaccine?

1. *Virtually every child will get rotavirus.* Without the vaccine, all children will experience fever, vomiting, and diarrhea associated with a rotavirus infection some time before five years of age.

2. *Some children with rotavirus are hospitalized.* Every year, many children are hospitalized with rotavirus. In fact, before the rotavirus vaccine, hospital wards were filled with children dehydrated by the disease every winter. Collectively, American parents could expect four hundred thousand visits to the doctor's office, two hundred thousand visits to the emergency department, seventy thousand hospitalizations, and sixty deaths caused by rotavirus infections annually.

3. *A limited window of opportunity exists for getting is vaccine.* The first dose must be given before fifteen weeks of age and the last dose no later than eight months of age.

4. *The vaccine is safe.*

ROTAVIRUS: OTHER THINGS YOU MIGHT HAVE WONDERED ABOUT

Rotavirus Disease in Other Countries

Rotavirus infects virtually every child in the world. In low- and middle-income countries, about 75 of 100 children get their first infection before one year of age. Before the rotavirus vaccine, every year, rotavirus infections were estimated to cause twenty-five million doctors' visits, two million hospitalizations, and more than five hundred thousand deaths. Due to the introduction of rotavirus vaccine in many countries, by 2013, annual global deaths were estimated to have declined to about 215,000. Most deaths from rotavirus are the result of dehydration and occur in countries where medical care is limited. By 2013, almost half of rotavirus fatalities occurred in just four countries: India, Nigeria, Pakistan, and Democratic Republic of the Congo. Groups involved in global health continue working to introduce the rotavirus vaccine in countries where it is needed. To monitor progress, visit the website of the Pan American Health Organization (PAHO): https://www.paho.org/en/topics/rotavirus.

Rotavirus: Additional Resources

ONLINE INFORMATION

"Living Proof Project: Rotavirus Vaccine's Remarkable Impact": https://www.youtube.com/watch?v=HwUicj5P6i8

"A Look at Each Vaccine: Rotavirus Vaccine": https://www.chop.edu /centers-programs/vaccine-education-center/vaccine-details/rotavirus -vaccine

"Rotavirus": https://www.vaccineinformation.org/diseases/rotavirus/

"Rotavirus Vaccine": https://www.voicesforvaccines.org/vaccine -information/rotovirus/

"Rotavirus: What You Should Know": https://media.chop.edu/data /files/pdfs/vaccine-education-center-rotavirus.pdf

PHOTOS

"Rotavirus Photos": https://www.vaccineinformation.org/photos/rotavirus/

PERSONAL EXPERIENCES

"Parents PACK Personal Stories – Rotavirus": https://www.chop.edu /centers-programs/parents-pack/personal-stories/rotavirus

"Story Gallery": https://www.shotbyshot.org/story-gallery/ (search "rotavirus")

"Unprotected People Stories: Rotavirus": https://www.immunize.org /clinical/vaccine-confidence/unprotected-people/topic/rotavirus/

HAEMOPHILUS INFLUENZAE TYPE B (Hib)

HIB: THE DISEASE

Although it might sound like influenza, *Haemophilus influenzae* type b (Hib) isn't related to the virus that causes influenza pandemics. In fact, before the Hib vaccine, Hib was the most common cause of bacterial meningitis in children less than five years old and, as a consequence, the most common cause of acquired cognitive developmental delay.

What Is Haemophilus influenzae *Type b?*

Hib is a bacterium that, before the availability of a vaccine, caused twenty-five thousand cases of severe disease in young children in the United States every year, specifically, meningitis, bloodstream infections, sepsis, joint infections, pneumonia, and epiglottitis, a disease that causes suffocation.

ONE PERSON'S STORY

"I was overcome with guilt as I watched the ventilator pump oxygen into Sarah's tiny lungs. In addition to large doses of antibiotics, the nurses injected her IV with a drug that would temporarily paralyze her, preventing her from becoming restless and dislodging the airway she so desperately needed. I was familiar with the drug, so I knew Sarah could still feel every poke and procedure, but was unable to respond. Knowing that I could have prevented her from going through such torture was almost unbearable."

Source: Archer, Peggy. "A Mother's Experience with *Haemophilus Influenzae* Type b." Immunize.org. August 21, 1998. https://www.immunize .org/clinical/vaccine-confidence/unprotected-people/story/a-mothers -experience-with-haemophilus-influenzae-type-b/.

Before the Hib vaccine was first made available in the early 1990s, as many as 4 of 100 people carried the bacteria on the lining of their nose and throat. Although most weren't sick, they could still transmit Hib to others by coughing or sneezing.

Diseases caused by Hib occur most commonly between September and December and between March and May. Children less than two years old are at the highest risk of infection.

DID YOU KNOW?

More than 90 of 100 cases of Hib disease occur in children less than five years old.

THINGS TO DO

Almost all mothers have antibodies against Hib that pass through the placenta to the baby before birth. Unfortunately, during the first six months of life, these antibodies fade away. Therefore, children need to be fully immune by the time they are six months old when they become most susceptible to the disease.

What Are the Symptoms of Hib?

When Hib bacteria get into the bloodstream, they can cause several types of infection:

- *Meningitis*: Hib most commonly infects the lining of the brain and spinal cord. More than 50 of 100 children with Hib have meningitis. Symptoms of meningitis include fever, confusion, stiff neck, and headache. About three to four of 100 people in high-income countries and 20 to 60 of 100 people in low- and middle-income countries die from Hib meningitis. Up to 30 of 100 survivors suffer hearing loss, seizures, decreased motor skills, cognitive developmental delays, or other forms of brain damage. Before the Hib vaccine,

Hib was the most common cause of acquired cognitive developmental delay.

- *Epiglottitis*: Hib is unique among bacteria in its capacity to infect the epiglottis, a membrane that covers the voice box and protects it during swallowing. When the epiglottis swells, it can cause difficulty breathing and be life threatening. Once infected, the epiglottis blocks the windpipe, causing suffocation and death. About one in 10 people with Hib develop epiglottitis.
- *Bloodstream infections*: Occur in about one of 12 or 13 people with Hib.
- *Arthritis or joint swelling*: Before the Hib vaccine, Hib was far and away the bacteria most likely to cause bacterial (septic) arthritis. About one in 25 people with Hib develop this condition.
- *Skin infections*: Hib is a common cause of skin infection, called cellulitis, occurring in about one in 20 people with Hib. It typically affects the cheeks, the area around the eyes, and other parts of the face.
- *Pneumonia*: About one in 10 people with Hib develop pneumonia (inflammation of the lungs).
- *Other conditions*: Occasionally, Hib infections can cause other conditions, including ear infections, sinus infections, bronchitis (infection of the large breathing tubes), and inflammation of the muscles associated with the heart, trachea, or a tube associated with the testicles (called the epididymis).

DID YOU KNOW?

Before 1990, every big city hospital had an "epiglottis team" designed to take children with epiglottitis quickly and quietly to the operating room so that they wouldn't become agitated before their airway could be opened. Agitation can cause children with epiglottitis to suffocate on the spot. Few diseases are more frightening.

HIB: THE VACCINE
What Is the Hib Vaccine?

The Hib vaccine is made from the complex sugar (polysaccharide) that coats the bacteria. The polysaccharide is attached to a "helper protein" that allows the immune system to generate a stronger, longer-lasting immune response than if the polysaccharide were given alone.

Three Hib vaccines are currently available in the United States: ActHIB, PedvaxHIB, and Hiberix. They differ in the helper protein used.

Who Should Get the Hib Vaccine?

The AAP and the CDC recommend that all infants get the Hib vaccine at two months, four months, six months, and between twelve and fifteen months of age, unless they get the PedvaxHIB vaccine, which requires only three doses (at two months, four months, and between twelve and fifteen months of age) because it induces a better response after the first dose than the other Hib vaccines.

The Hib vaccine is sometimes given as part of a combination vaccine to reduce the number of shots a baby gets in a single visit. Both Pentacel and Vaxelis include Hib (See "Combination Vaccines" section for more details.).

Children who do not start their vaccines in the first six months of life will get fewer doses depending on their age and which product they receive, and those who do not get vaccinated against Hib by five years of age will not receive this vaccine at all since most Hib infections occur before that age.

Does the Hib Vaccine Work?

In the United States, the Hib vaccine has virtually eliminated Hib infections—which once afflicted more than twenty thousand children every year. No vaccine has had a greater impact on today's practicing pediatrician.

DID YOU KNOW?

Unfortunately, decreases in vaccine use could quickly result in the return of this infection. Outbreaks in Minnesota in 2008 and Pennsylvania in 2009 caused four deaths. Since 2010, cases for which the type of *Haemophilus influenzae* could be determined have averaged around a dozen cases caused by type b per year in the United States.

Who Should Avoid or Delay Getting the Hib Vaccine?

Children less than six weeks old should not get the Hib vaccine, nor should children who have had a severe allergic reaction to previous doses. Children with a moderate or severe illness should delay getting the vaccine until they are feeling better; however, children with mild illnesses (such as ear infections or diarrhea) can still get vaccinated.

What Are the Side Effects of the Hib Vaccine?

About 15 of 100 recipients will experience pain, redness, or swelling at the injection site. Some babies will be irritable, experience loss of appetite, or develop a low-grade fever. These symptoms usually go away in about a day.

Why Get the Hib Vaccine?

1. *Hib is still around.* Every year a small number of children are infected with Hib in the United States. In 2008 and 2009, four children died from Hib because their parents chose not to vaccinate them.

2. *Infants and young children are the most susceptible.* Before the vaccine was available, about 60 of 100 infections occurred in infants between six and eleven months of age. If infants are vaccinated before six months, when maternal antibodies are still somewhat protective, they can fight the disease with their own immune systems after the maternal antibodies fade.

3. *Unvaccinated or incompletely vaccinated children are at higher risk of disease.* In studies, infants too young to be immunized with the first three doses (i.e., those less than six months of age) accounted for almost half of infections. Of those infected at an age older than six months, most had not received the vaccine at all or had not received all the recommended doses.

4. *Vaccine use decreases the number of carriers in the population.* As more infants are vaccinated, fewer will have Hib bacteria in their nose and throat. This is important because they will be less likely to pass the bacteria to others, especially those who cannot be vaccinated (see "Is It My Social Responsibility to Get Vaccinated?").

5. *The vaccine is safe.* Although some mild side effects may occur, the vaccine is safe.

HIB: OTHER THINGS YOU MIGHT HAVE WONDERED ABOUT
Hib and Influenza: Are They Related?

People may wonder whether *Haemophilus influenzae* type b and influenza are related because of the similarity of their names; however, they are different. Hib is a bacterium, and influenza is a virus. The similarity in names is historical.

Influenza was known as an illness well before its cause was understood. Following the influenza pandemic in 1889, a scientist named Richard Pfeiffer isolated Hib bacteria from patients who were ill, so he thought it caused influenza. But it didn't. Influenza was later found to be caused by a virus, not a bacterium.

Hib: Additional Resources
ONLINE INFORMATION

"*Haemophilus influenzae* (Hib) Vaccine": https://www.voicesforvaccines
  .org/vaccine-information/hib/

"Hib (*Haemophilus influenzae* Type b)": https://www.vaccineinformation
  .org/diseases/hib/

"A Look at Each Vaccine: *Haemophilus Influenzae* Type b (Hib) Vaccine":
  https://www.chop.edu/centers-programs/vaccine-education-center
  /vaccine-details/haemophilus-influenzae-type-b-hib-vaccine

PHOTOS

"Hib Photos": https://www.vaccineinformation.org/photos/hib/

PERSONAL EXPERIENCES

"Story Gallery": https://www.shotbyshot.org/story-gallery/ (search "hib")
"Unprotected People Stories: Hib (*Haemophilus Influenzae* Type b)":
    https://www.immunize.org/clinical/vaccine-confidence/unprotected
    -people/topic/hib/

POLIO

POLIO: THE DISEASE

You've probably never seen someone with polio. Unfortunately, while the fear of polio is largely gone, the disease isn't. Polio transmission has yet to be stopped in Pakistan and Afghanistan, and outbreaks are common in several other countries. Because international travel is common, the polio vaccine continues to be recommended for all children in the United States.

The international spread of polio isn't just theoretical. In July 2022, an unvaccinated person was paralyzed by polio in New York. Because most people who get polio experience only mild illness or no symptoms at all, one case of paralytic polio indicates that the number of people infected with the virus is probably much higher. People infected with polio shed the virus in their saliva and feces. This is how the virus spreads from person to person, but it also means the virus can be found in wastewater. So to confirm wider exposure in New York during the fall of 2022, public health officials conducted wastewater sampling in and around the area where the individual lived, finding the virus in samples from several counties in the area.

What Is Polio?

Polio is caused by a virus found in the intestines of infected people, and it is spread easily by food, hands, and other objects that may find their way into a person's mouth. The virus spreads in saliva or after exposure to the feces of an infected person, such as after changing a diaper and not washing one's hands properly.

What Are the Symptoms of Polio?

People infected with polio suffer a range of symptoms:

- About 90 of 100 people with polio won't experience any symptoms, and, although contagious to others, they won't realize they're

infected. In the United States in 1950—five years before the first
polio vaccine became available—more than thirty-three thousand
people were paralyzed by polio, and three million were infected.
This meant that two of every one hundred people living in the
United States were infected in just one year.

• About six of 100 infected people will be mildly ill with symptoms
typical of other viral infections, such as sore throat, fever, nausea,
vomiting, abdominal pain, and constipation.

• About one of 100 people will experience severe disease, beginning
with flu-like symptoms, muscle aches, fever, sore throat, and vomiting. These individuals will either develop meningitis or paralytic
polio. The paralysis is characterized by a lack of tone and reflexes
in affected muscles. Before the polio vaccine, tens of thousands of
people were paralyzed, and thousands were killed by polio in the
United States every year.

ONE PERSON'S STORY

"The local doctor stopped by for a look. His comforting diagnosis—
a 'bug' compounded by physical exhaustion—made perfect sense.
Even the most severe polio cases can be mistaken for run-of-the-
mill influenza, until paralysis sets in. For [Franklin Delano] Roosevelt, however, a downward spiral had begun. His pain grew worse,
the fever lingered, and numbness spread to both legs. His skin was
so sensitive that he couldn't tolerate the feel of his pajamas or even
the rustle of a breeze."

Source: Oshinsky, David M. *Polio: An American Story*. New York: Oxford
University Press, 2005.

POLIO: THE VACCINE
What Is the Polio Vaccine?

The polio vaccine used in the United States today contains the
three known types of polio virus (types 1, 2, and 3). The vaccine is
made by growing polio viruses in monkey kidney cells, purifying

the viruses away from the cells, and then treating them with formaldehyde so that they can no longer reproduce and cause disease. Because the viruses can't replicate, the vaccine is referred to as the inactivated polio vaccine (IPV).

The first polio vaccine, made in 1955 by Jonas Salk, was similar to the one used today. It was the product of a massive nationwide effort spearheaded by President Franklin Delano Roosevelt, who had himself previously been affected by polio. Roosevelt urged citizens to send their dimes to the White House to help fund polio vaccine research as part of a fundraising campaign that became known as the March of Dimes. This effort led to a vaccine trial that included almost two million children—the largest test of a medical product in history.

DID YOU KNOW?

Franklin Delano Roosevelt's support of the March of Dimes is the reason he is pictured on the dime.

Jonas Salk wasn't the only researcher to make a polio vaccine. In 1961, a second vaccine, made by Albert Sabin, became available. Known as the oral polio vaccine (OPV), it was used in the United States from 1961 to 1998. Like the Salk vaccine, OPV contained polio virus types 1, 2, and 3. But unlike the Salk vaccine, which was completely inactivated with formaldehyde, the Sabin vaccine contained vaccine viruses weakened by growth in laboratory cells (see "How Are Vaccines Made?"). Sabin's vaccine offered several advantages over IPV. It was more economical to make, easier to use (given as drops by mouth rather than as a shot in the arm), and, because it reproduced in the intestines and was shed in the feces, could be spread from a vaccinated person to an unvaccinated person causing them also to become immune to the weakened virus (known as contact immunity).

Unfortunately, OPV also had one major drawback: in rare cases, the vaccine could itself cause polio. This could happen in vaccinated individuals or in those exposed through contact immunity. Before the United States switched back to IPV in 2000, every year about six to eight people were paralyzed by OPV. In these cases, known as vaccine-associated paralytic polio or VAPP, the vaccine virus had reverted to the dangerous form. By 1980, the only cases of paralytic polio occurring in the United States were those caused by the vaccine. For this reason, experts suggested going back to the inactivated version (see "Who Recommends Vaccines?"). Although OPV is no longer used in the United States, it is still used in some other countries.

Who Should Get the Polio Vaccine?

All children are recommended to receive four doses of the polio vaccine, given as a shot, at two months, four months, between six and eighteen months, and between four and six years of age. Children who do not get the vaccine as infants or who fall behind on their doses should still get four doses of IPV, each separated by at least four weeks.

Adults eighteen years of age and older are assumed to be protected against polio; however, the case of polio in New York in 2022 led some to question their immunity, particularly if they did not have vaccination records. In response, the CDC stated, "Unless there are specific reasons to believe they were not vaccinated, most adults who were born and raised in the United States can assume they were vaccinated for polio as children." However, if someone is unvaccinated or only partially vaccinated and they are at high risk due to travel, occupation, outbreak, or potential for exposure to someone who received OPV (e.g., parents of international adoptees), they should be vaccinated with IPV. If they were previously vaccinated and are at high risk, they can get one lifetime booster dose of IPV. Unvaccinated or partially vaccinated adults not at high risk should speak with their health care provider to determine whether they need any doses.

Does the Polio Vaccine Work?

About 95 of 100 infants will be protected against all three types of poliovirus after two doses of IPV, and 99 of 100 will be protected after three doses. The fourth dose is given to boost the immune response.

Who Should Avoid or Delay Getting the Polio Vaccine?

People who have had a severe allergic reaction to previous doses of the vaccine should not get additional doses. Those who are pregnant or mildly ill should delay vaccination until after delivery or recovery, respectively.

What Are the Side Effects of the Polio Vaccine?

The polio vaccine occasionally causes redness, tenderness, swelling, and pain at the injection site. The inactivated polio vaccine cannot cause polio.

Why Get the Polio Vaccine?

1. *Polio still exists in the world.* In 2016, only about fifty people worldwide were paralyzed by polio. By 2020, that number had risen to almost two thousand. Because international travel is common, polio has been spreading. Maybe someday polio, like smallpox, will be eliminated from the world, and we can stop using the polio vaccine. But that day has not yet arrived.
2. *Paralytic polio can be devastating.* While most people experience relatively minor disease, many do not.
3. *Polio infection can lead to postpolio syndrome later in life.* Some people with polio will experience a recurrence of muscle weakness and pain later in life. Known as post-polio syndrome, the condition most often affects those who had paralytic polio infections in childhood and typically appears fifteen to forty years after the initial infection.
4. *The vaccine is safe.* Side effects are minor and relatively uncommon.

POLIO: OTHER THINGS YOU MIGHT HAVE WONDERED ABOUT

Eradicating Polio

The only disease that has ever successfully been eliminated from the face of the globe is smallpox. One of the goals of the World Health Organization is to rid the world of polio through efforts coordinated by a coalition of international partners known as the Global Polio Eradication Initiative (https://polioeradication .org/). While efforts have been largely successful, work remains:

- Two of the three types of polio (types 2 and 3) have been eliminated, but vaccine-derived type 2 poliovirus continues to cause infections. *Vaccine-derived* refers to virus that has reverted to its infectious form after being delivered in the OPV vaccine. The spread of vaccine-derived type 2 poliovirus in New York City in 2022 is probably the tip of the iceberg. This "vaccine-derived" paralytic virus is yet another reason to give the polio vaccine in countries where the "wild type" or natural virus has been eliminated.
- Polio transmission has never been interrupted in two countries (Pakistan and Afghanistan), down from 125 countries in 1988. Small outbreaks continue to occur in countries around the world.
- Annual global cases of polio are extremely low but have started to creep up in the last couple of years, going from about fifty cases of paralysis in 2016 to almost two thousand in 2020.

The Global Polio Eradication Initiative has developed a new strategic plan for 2022 to 2026 to eradicate this devastating disease once and for all. To learn more, visit their website: https://polioeradication.org/gpei-strategy-2022-2026.

Post-polio Syndrome

About 30 of 100 people who experienced paralytic polio will have a recurrence later in life. Known as post-polio syndrome, symptoms include muscle pain, a worsening of residual muscle weakness, and new muscle weakness or paralysis.

Polio: Additional Resources

ONLINE INFORMATION

"2022 NY Polio Case: Why and What Does It Mean?": https://www
.chop.edu/news/2022-ny-polio-case-why-and-what-does-it-mean

"A Look at Each Vaccine: Polio Vaccine": https://www.chop.edu/centers
-programs/vaccine-education-center/vaccine-details/polio-vaccine

"Polio": https://www.vaccineinformation.org/diseases/polio/

"Polio Vaccine": https://www.voicesforvaccines.org/vaccine-information
/polio/

PHOTOS

"Polio Photos": https://www.vaccineinformation.org/photos/polio/

PERSONAL EXPERIENCES

"Parents PACK Personal Stories – Polio": http://www.chop.edu/service
/parents-possessing-accessing-communicating-knowledge-about
-vaccines/sharing-personal-stories/sharing-personal-stories-polio
.html

"Unprotected People Stories: Polio": https://www.immunize.org/clinical
/vaccine-confidence/unprotected-people/topic/polio/

SUPPORT GROUPS

The Polio Survivors Network provides information and support
to polio survivors, post-polio groups, families, and caregivers.
Although this group is headquartered in Pennsylvania, they work
with individuals and groups from across the country and around
the world: https://www.polionetwork.org.

Post-Polio Health International supports polio survivors and shares
information about the effects of polio experienced later in life:
https://post-polio.org.

BOOKS

Nichols, Janice Flood. *Twin Voices: A Memoir of Polio, the Forgotten
Killer.* Self-published, iUniverse, 2007.

Offit, Paul A. *The Cutter Incident: How America's First Polio Vaccine Led to the Growing Vaccine Crisis*. New Haven, CT: Yale University Press, 2005.

Oshinsky, David M. *Polio: An American Story*. New York: Oxford University Press, 2005.

Wunsch, Hannah. *The Autumn Ghost: How the Battle Against a Polio Epidemic Revolutionized Modern Medical Care*. Vancouver: Greystone, 2023.

INFLUENZA

INFLUENZA: THE DISEASE

Swine flu. Bird flu. Seasonal flu. Influenza. H1N1. Nasal-spray vaccine. Flu shot. Live virus. Killed virus. Epidemics. Pandemics. Influenza is so unique and so unpredictable that public health officials often quip, "If you want job security in public health, work on influenza."

Although unpredictable, influenza is quite interesting. First, infections aren't restricted to people: the virus infects a wide range of animals. Second, the virus changes enough from one year to the next that a yearly vaccine is required. Indeed, sometimes the virus changes significantly as it travels from one hemisphere to the next. Third, several approaches to vaccines have been successful, making various options available.

What Is Influenza?

Influenza is a virus that infects people as well as several species of animals, including chickens, pigs, horses, dogs, cats, aquatic birds, and sea mammals. Influenza infections most commonly occur between November and May in the United States. The virus is transmitted from one person to another by coughing or sneezing; however, if people touch contaminated surfaces and then touch their eyes, nose, or mouth, they can also be infected. Several types of influenza viruses have been identified: types A, B, C, and D. Type D infects cattle and occasionally other animals but not people.

Influenza A viruses are the ones we need to worry about most because they infect numerous types of animals, are passed between species, and lead to epidemics (widespread disease in a certain geographic region) and pandemics (worldwide epidemics). Influenza A viruses are further identified by their two surface proteins: hemagglutinin (H) and neuraminidase (N). Hemagglutinin helps influenza virus attach to cells, and neuraminidase allows influenza virus to escape infected cells. Eighteen H types and 11 N types have been identified; those that most commonly infect people are H1N1 and H3N2.

Influenza B viruses can also infect people and make them quite ill, but they don't cause pandemics. Similarly, influenza C virus infections are limited to people and pigs and don't typically cause severe disease.

DID YOU KNOW?

The bird flu strain that spread from chickens to people in Asia beginning in 1997 was H5N1. Although many scientists and public health officials feared that this strain would cause a pandemic, it didn't. Since then, H5N1 outbreaks have periodically occurred in bird populations around the world, and, in a few isolated cases, people who were close to or working with infected birds got the virus. However, these strains had not gained the ability to spread from person to person. In 2022 and 2023, H5N1 was detected in wild birds, commercial poultry, and several wild mammals across the United States. Although the virus was detected in more than seven thousand wild birds and almost fifty-eight million poultry by early July 2023, only one person was diagnosed with H5N1 during that period, and that individual had worked with infected poultry. In March 2024, H5N1 was detected in a large number of dairy cattle, a few cats, and one person who had worked with infected dairy cattle.

THINGS TO DO

Influenza transmission can be reduced by washing or disinfecting hands frequently and thoroughly, sneezing and coughing into a bent arm, and staying home when ill. However, because we can't be sure those around us practice these measures and because none is foolproof, a vaccine is still the best way to protect yourself and your family.

What Are the Symptoms of Influenza?

People with influenza sometimes have mild symptoms. More commonly, however, the disease "knocks you out," and it often takes several weeks to recover and regain one's energy. About half those with influenza will have classic symptoms that can include:

- Sudden onset of fever (101–102°F) that occurs so suddenly people remember the exact hour they became ill
- Muscle aches
- Sore throat
- Cough
- Headache
- Runny nose
- Burning sensation in the chest
- Eye pain
- Sensitivity to light

Complications of influenza can include:

- Pneumonia caused by influenza virus or by bacteria that take advantage of lungs weakened by influenza
- Myocarditis (an inflammation of the heart muscle)
- Encephalitis (an inflammation of the brain)

People at highest risk of complications include those younger than two and older than sixty-five years of age; people with chronic conditions of the lungs, heart, or kidneys; residents of nursing homes or other long-term care facilities; and pregnant people. Every year thousands to tens of thousands of people die of influenza in the United States; the average annual death rate from influenza is about thirty-six thousand. This is about the same number of annual deaths attributed to car accidents (about thirty-five thousand to forty-seven thousand) and firearms (about thirty-six thousand to forty-nine thousand).

Pregnant people are at increased risk of complications from influenza for three reasons. First, they have an increased volume of blood, which can seep out a little at the lining of the lungs, making lungs "wetter" and more susceptible to pneumonia. Second, their immune response is somewhat suppressed so that the fetus is not perceived by the mother's immune system as foreign. Third, as the growing fetus pushes up on the lungs, it becomes increasingly more difficult to breathe deeply.

People are often surprised to learn that children die from influenza each year. Some of these children are at increased risk because of other health conditions, but many are previously healthy children whose influenza infection was severe. However, COVID-19 showed us that we could prevent most, if not all, deaths from influenza. During the 2019–2020 influenza season, about two hundred children died from influenza. On the other hand, during the influenza seasons that occurred during the COVID-19 pandemic (2020–2021 and 2021–2022), one child and forty-six children, respectively, died from influenza. In the 2022–2023 season, as life began to return to normal, the number of children who died from influenza increased again to about 160. Vaccination, staying home when ill, and preventive measures like covering coughs and frequently washing hands can limit the ability of influenza to wreak havoc on our children.

"At the hospital, Breanne's temperature rose to 107°F. Her temperature was brought down by doctors in the emergency room, but

Breanne had to be transferred to another hospital for more intensive care. A special life-support machine was needed as the virus began to attack Breanne's heart and brain stem. However, after being transferred to yet another hospital, doctors told Breanne's parents that the damage to her young body was too extensive. There was nothing the life-support machine could do. Breanne died in her mother's arms on December 23, 2003, from influenza A."

Source: "Breanne Palmer." Families Fighting Flu. Accessed August 10, 2023, at https://www.familiesfightingflu.org/family-story/the-palmer -family/.

INFLUENZA: THE VACCINE

What Is the Influenza Vaccine?

Several types of influenza vaccines are available.

Inactivated influenza vaccine. This version of the influenza vaccine has been available since 1945 and is given as a shot. After the virus is grown in eggs, it is purified and treated with a chemical that completely inactivates the virus so that it cannot cause disease. Several inactivated flu vaccines are available, and most can be used in anyone six months of age and older. Examples include Afluria, Fluarix, and Fluzone. Two versions are specifically designed for those aged sixty-five years and older. These either have higher quantities of antigen (the part of the virus that our immune systems make a response to), or they include an adjuvant that helps generate stronger immunity. Fluzone High-Dose is an example of the former, and Fluad is an example of the latter.

Live, weakened influenza vaccine. First available in 2003, this version is given as a nasal spray. It offers a great example of scientific progress. The influenza virus was adapted in the lab so that it can grow at temperatures commonly found in the nose (around 89.6°F) but not those found inside the body (around 98.6°F). When the vaccine is given, the virus can reproduce enough in the nose to cause immunity but not enough to cause illness. Like the inactivated vaccine viruses, those used in this vaccine are grown in eggs. FluMist is an example of this type of influenza vaccine. It can be given to healthy people between two and forty-nine years of age.

Cell-culture-based influenza vaccine. The vaccine viruses in this version are grown in mammalian cells, purified and inactivated. The vaccine is given as a shot, and because of how it is produced, it does not contain egg proteins or antibiotics. Flucelvax is an example of this type; it can be given to anyone six months of age or older.

Recombinant influenza vaccine. This version is made by adding the gene for hemagglutinin (one of the influenza virus surface proteins) into an insect virus. As the insect virus reproduces, the hemagglutinin protein is also produced. The purified-protein vaccine is given as a shot. It does not contain any egg proteins or antibiotics. Flublok is an example of this type; it can be given to those eighteen years of age and older.

For several years, seasonal influenza vaccines have contained four influenza viruses—two type B viruses and two type A viruses, usually an H_1N_1 strain and an H_3N_2 strain. However, starting in the 2024-2025 influenza season, annual vaccines will only contain three influenza viruses. One of the type B influenza viruses has not been circulating since March 2020, so the vaccines no longer need to protect against it. The decision regarding which strains are used for U.S. vaccines each year is made between January and March and is based on monitoring the influenza strains circulating in the Southern Hemisphere. The hard part for public health officials is waiting as long as possible to get the most representative strains but not so long that the vaccine isn't ready in time.

DID YOU KNOW?

Because influenza virus changes rapidly and because the vaccine takes several months to produce, some years the vaccine more closely matches circulating influenza viruses than others. Unfortunately, when people get the vaccine and still get influenza, they lose confidence in the vaccine program. However, it is important to remember that some immunity is better than no immunity, so a vaccine that is only a partial match is better than none.

THINGS TO DO

Influenza vaccines are offered each fall; however, cases usually peak in January or February and can occur throughout the spring, so people can still get the influenza vaccine even after the season has started.

DID YOU KNOW?

The novel H1N1 influenza vaccine used during the fall of 2009 to protect people from pandemic influenza was made in the same way that seasonal influenza vaccines are made. In fact, if the pandemic strain had emerged a few months earlier, it would likely have been part of the seasonal vaccine rather than a second, separate influenza vaccine. The 2010–2011 version of the influenza vaccine contained the 2009 H1N1 pandemic strain along with two other influenza strains.

Who Should Get the Influenza Vaccine?

Influenza vaccines are recommended for everyone six months of age and older. Most people require only a single dose; however, any child less than nine years old who is getting an influenza vaccine for the first time should get two doses separated by one month. Even if your child receives the first dose late in the season, it is important to go back for the second dose one month later. If this doesn't happen, two doses will still be needed the following year.

Adults sixty-five years of age and older should try to get one of the versions that has been designed to enhance immunity in this age group, such as Fluad, Flublok, or Fluzone High-Dose; however, if one of those is not available, older adults should get whichever version they can get at the time since some immunity is better than none.

Who Should Avoid or Delay Getting the Influenza Vaccine?

Infants younger than six months of age and people who have had a severe allergic reaction to a previous dose of influenza vaccine or a vaccine component shouldn't get this vaccine. Importantly, people with egg allergies can get the influenza vaccine, and most can get any version because even the versions grown in eggs have such tiny amounts of egg protein that they will not cause a reaction. However, people with severe egg allergies now also have the option to receive versions made without the use of eggs.

Several groups should not receive the live, weakened, nasal-spray influenza vaccine (FluMist):

- Children less than two years old
- Adults fifty years of age or older
- Pregnant people
- Those who are immune compromised
- Those on long-term aspirin therapy
- Those who have recently taken certain antiviral medications (check with your health care provider for specific situations)
- Children between the ages of two and four years who have been diagnosed with asthma or who have had a wheezing episode in the previous twelve months
- People with cochlear implants or cerebrospinal fluid leaks
- People without a functional spleen
- Caregivers or close contacts of people whose immune-compromising condition requires them to be in a protected environment (however, people in this group can get vaccinated if they will be away from the affected individual for at least seven days after vaccination)

People with moderate or severe illness should delay getting any influenza vaccine until they are feeling better, and those who developed Guillain-Barré syndrome (GBS) within six weeks of a previous dose of influenza vaccine should talk with their health care provider. Importantly, a history of GBS alone is not a reason to forgo influenza vaccination.

Those five years and older who have asthma or a condition that increases their risk from influenza should discuss the relative risks and benefits of getting the nasal influenza vaccine compared with the shot with their health care provider.

Does the Influenza Vaccine Work?

In most years, about 65 of 100 people given the vaccine will be protected from getting very sick from influenza. Some years are better than others when it comes to how well influenza vaccines protect against the circulating strains because of how quickly the virus changes.

What Are the Side Effects of the Influenza Vaccine?

Influenza vaccines are safe but may cause a few side effects. The influenza shot causes pain, redness, and swelling at the injection site in about 18 of 100 people who get it. About 10 of every 100 people could experience headache or low-grade fever. In very rare cases, people will have an allergic reaction such as hives (about one person of ten thousand), and an even smaller number may develop GBS (about one person of one million).

The nasal-spray vaccine causes cough, runny nose, and congestion in about 50 to 60 of 100 people who get it, and about seven to 10 of 100 people will have a sore throat. Some younger children with asthma might also have a mild bout of wheezing.

DID YOU KNOW?

Some people are concerned about developing Guillain-Barré syndrome (GBS) after getting the influenza vaccine. GBS is a disorder that affects the lining of the nerves, causing temporary and occasionally permanent paralysis. A swine flu vaccine distributed in 1976 was found to cause GBS in one of one hundred thousand

(*continued on next page*)

(*continued from previous page*)

people who got it; however, studies of subsequent influenza vaccines, including the 2009 novel H1N1 vaccine, have found instances of GBS after influenza vaccination to be extremely rare—about one case per one million doses. While that may feel like too big of a risk for some, context is important: influenza infections can also cause GBS, and the rate of GBS resulting from natural influenza infection is about seventeen cases per one million infections. So, the vaccine actually reduces a person's risk of GBS!

If a person developed GBS within six weeks of getting an influenza vaccine, they have a "precaution" for receiving influenza vaccine, meaning they should talk with their health care provider about the relative risks and benefits of receiving the vaccine. However, if a person had GBS, but it did not occur within six weeks of getting an influenza vaccine, they do not have the same precaution. They are recommended to get influenza vaccine, like most other people in the population.

Why Get the Influenza Vaccine?

1. *Influenza infections are common.* Every year in the United States, two hundred thousand people are hospitalized and thousands to tens of thousands die from influenza. Although hospitalizations and deaths from influenza occur most commonly in high-risk groups, every year between fifty and 150 previously healthy children die from the disease. Because there is no way of knowing who these children will be, all benefit from receiving the vaccine.

2. *Influenza spreads easily.* After visiting her child's elementary school classroom, a mom once said, "A child sneezes where a child pleases." Indeed, this is why children are so good at spreading influenza—to their grandparents, to younger siblings, to their pregnant mothers, and to many others who may be at increased risk of getting severely ill.

3. *Infections with influenza can lead to other infections.* When people are ill with influenza, their immune systems are weakened, so they are at increased risk of getting other infections, including bacterial infections that can lead to pneumonia. Infections caused by some of these "opportunistic" bacteria are vaccine preventable, such as Hib and pneumococcus; others aren't. Those sixty-five years of age and older are particularly susceptible to severe outcomes, particularly pneumonia, either from the influenza infection or a secondary bacterial infection.

4. *The vaccine is safe.* Influenza vaccines are safe, causing only minimal side effects.

INFLUENZA: OTHER THINGS YOU MIGHT HAVE WONDERED ABOUT

Chickens, Pigs, and Pandemics

Pigs are typically infected with pig strains of influenza virus; however, on occasion they can also be infected with influenza viruses from birds (like chickens) or people. When this happens, the viruses can exchange genetic material and make "new" influenza viruses. These new influenza viruses can die, spread to other pigs, or spread to people, occasionally causing pandemics.

Making the Influenza Vaccine

Every year, public health officials monitor the strains of influenza circulating throughout the world, and between January and March, they determine which are most likely to cause disease in the United States. After the strains are chosen, vaccine manufacturers begin production. The strains of influenza must be grown, tested for safety, packaged, and distributed within six to eight months so vaccine doses are available by early fall.

If the influenza strains that were circulating in the winter stay about the same, the vaccine will be a good match; however, if the virus changes significantly or a new virus emerges, the vaccine may not work as well. Importantly, even in years when the vaccine is not a good match, tens of thousands of hospitalizations and thousands of deaths are still averted. For example, the influenza vaccines used in the 2014–2015 season were the least effective in recent years, protecting only about one in five people who got vaccinated. However, about forty thousand fewer people were hospitalized, and about 3,700 fewer people died as a result of getting vaccinated that season.

Hopefully, we will eventually have influenza vaccines that protect against parts of the virus less subject to change, so that we will have vaccines that are more consistently effective. But in the meantime, some protection is better than none. So, getting an annual influenza vaccine, which is safe and at least somewhat effective, is the more prudent choice.

Flu Versus "the Flu" (Do I Really Have Influenza?)

"I have the flu," is a common statement but not always an accurate one. Many respiratory viruses circulating during the winter, such as parainfluenza virus, respiratory syncytial virus (RSV), adenovirus, and rhinoviruses, are often called "the flu" when they are not. As a result, vaccinated people often think the vaccine didn't work when, in reality, they had some other infection. The influenza vaccine will not prevent other respiratory illnesses common at the same time of the year.

Influenza: Additional Resources

ONLINE INFORMATION

"Can a Flu Vaccine Give Me the Flu?": https://www.chop.edu/centers
-programs/vaccine-education-center/video/can-flu-vaccine-give
-you-flu

"Flu Vaccine: What's in the Vial?": https://media.chop.edu/data/files
/pdfs/flu-whats-in-the-vial-infographic.pdf"Influenza":https://media
.chop.edu/data/files/pdfs/vec-influenza-infographic.pdf

"How Are Strains of Influenza Chosen for the Annual Vaccine?":
https://www.chop.edu/video/how-are-strains-influenza-chosen
-annual-vaccine

"Influenza (Flu)": http://www.flu.gov/

"Influenza (Flu)": https://www.vaccineinformation.org/diseases/influenza/

"Influenza (Flu) Vaccine": https://www.voicesforvaccines.org/vaccine
-information/influenza/

"Influenza: What You Should Know": https://media.chop.edu/data
/files/pdfs/vaccine-education-center-influenza.pdf

"A Look at Each Vaccine: Influenza Vaccine": https://www.chop
.edu/centers-programs/vaccine-education-center/vaccine-details
/influenza-vaccine

"Why Doesn't the Influenza Vaccine Work for More than One Year?":
https://www.chop.edu/centers-programs/vaccine-education-center
/video/why-doesnt-influenza-vaccine-work-more-one-year

PHOTOS

"Influenza Photos": https://www.vaccineinformation.org/photos
/influenza/

PERSONAL EXPERIENCES

"Family Stories": https://www.familiesfightingflu.org/family-stories/

"Parents PACK Personal Stories – Influenza": https://www.chop.edu
/centers-programs/parents-pack/personal-stories/influenza

"Story Gallery": https://www.shotbyshot.org/story-gallery (search
"influenza")

"Unprotected People Stories: Influenza": http://www.immunize.org
/reports/influenza.asp

SUPPORT GROUPS

Families Fighting Flu was started by families whose lives were
changed forever when their children suffered and died from influenza. Visit their website to learn more about how families are
affected and what the group is doing to make sure that other children don't suffer this disease: http://www.familiesfightingflu.org.

BOOKS

Barry, John M. *The Great Influenza: The Story of the Deadliest Pandemic in History*. New York: Penguin, 2004.

Sipress, Alan. *The Fatal Strain: On the Trail of Avian Flu and the Coming Pandemic*. New York: Viking, 2009.

COVID-19

COVID-19: THE DISEASE

At the end of 2019, a novel coronavirus spread throughout the city of Wuhan, China, and then throughout the world. The virus was called SARS-CoV-2, which stands for "severe acute respiratory syndrome-coronavirus-2." By early 2024, the virus had killed about seven million people worldwide. Fortunately, by the end of 2020, vaccines were available to prevent severe infection, and antiviral medicines were available to treat it.

What Is COVID-19?

COVID-19, the disease caused by SARS-CoV-2, stands for "coronavirus disease-2019." This was the third coronavirus pandemic to appear in the last twenty years. The first, SARS-1, appeared in 2002. The second, MERS ("Middle East respiratory syndrome"), appeared in 2012, and the third, SARS-CoV-2, appeared in 2019. SARS-1 and SARS-CoV-2 first appeared in China. MERS first appeared in Saudi Arabia.

DID YOU KNOW?

In 2023, two-thirds of the American public believed that SARS-CoV-2 virus was either intentionally or accidentally created in a scientific laboratory in Wuhan, China. However, genetic evidence of samples taken from the western section of the Huanan Seafood Wholesale Market in Wuhan proved that the virus had been transmitted from animals to humans (in what is known as a spillover event), most likely from a bat coronavirus that infected another animal, probably a raccoon dog that was sold at the market, allowing it to infect people.

THINGS TO DO

When SARS-CoV-2 first entered the United States at the beginning of 2020, it was unclear exactly how it was transmitted from person to person. Early on, public health officials knew that it was transmitted by small droplets from the mouth after talking, sneezing, or coughing. But they worried that it could also be spread by touching an item that someone with COVID-19 had touched. So, people were told to wash surfaces, wash their hands, and wash items purchased at grocery stores. However, it soon became clear that all of this washing was unnecessary. But, taking precautions to diminish the spread of respiratory infections, like staying home when ill and covering coughs and sneezes, can help decrease the spread of COVID-19. Vaccines, however, afford the best protection because they generate virus-specific immunity, compared with other precautions, which are helpful but less specific.

What Are the Symptoms of COVID-19?

People with COVID-19 typically have mild symptoms, such as cough, congestion, runny nose, low-grade fever, joint pain, muscle pain, and headache. These symptoms typically resolve in a few days.

SARS-CoV-2 virus can also infect the lungs, causing severe and occasionally fatal pneumonia. Severe disease usually occurs in high-risk groups:

- People over sixty-five years of age
- People with certain medical conditions, such as chronic heart, lung, or kidney disease
- People who are immune compromised
- Pregnant people

DID YOU KNOW?

Pregnant people are two to three times more likely to be hospitalized, require intensive care, or die from COVID-19 than people of the same age who aren't pregnant. This is why it is critical that people receive a COVID-19 vaccine during every pregnancy.

ONE PERSON'S STORY

"In late 2021, Chris Crouch had a decision to make. His wife, Diana, who was 20 weeks pregnant, was in the intensive care unit and on a ventilator, struggling with COVID-19.

Neither Chris nor his wife had been vaccinated, even though a vaccine was available. Diana was placed on a heart-lung machine, which offered a 50 percent chance of survival. On Nov. 10, 2021, when the baby boy was 31-weeks' gestation, doctors delivered him by Caesarean section. He weighed 4 pounds and 12 ounces. Just before Christmas, on Dec. 23, 2021, Diana returned home. She still required an oxygen tank. But she was alive, and so was her baby."

Source: Cha, Ariana Eunjung. "Chris Crouch Was Anti-vaccine. Now His Pregnant Wife had COVID, and He Faced a Terrible Choice." *Washington Post*. February 14, 2022. https://www.washingtonpost.com /health/2022/02/14/unvaccinated-pregnant-mom-covid-strokes-texas/.

COVID-19: THE VACCINE
What Is the COVID-19 Vaccine?

The first two vaccines to prevent COVID-19 were authorized in December 2020. Produced by Pfizer and Moderna, both were made using a novel vaccine technology called messenger RNA (mRNA).

While using mRNA as a vaccine was novel, our bodies process mRNA every day. This is because mRNA is a blueprint that teaches our cells how to make proteins. In the case of these two COVID-19 vaccines, the protein was the spike protein that sits on the surface of SARS-CoV-2 virus. After our cells make the SARS-CoV-2 spike protein, our immune system makes antibodies against it, preventing the virus from infecting our cells when the antibodies bind to it during future encounters. Because the virus can't infect our cells, it can't cause disease.

In February 2021, the second type of COVID-19 vaccine became available. This one was made by Janssen/Johnson & Johnson (Janssen/J&J). Instead of using mRNA, the gene (made of DNA) that serves as a blueprint for the SARS-CoV-2 spike protein was added to a different virus. That virus, called adenovirus type 26, couldn't reproduce, so it couldn't cause disease. But it could enter cells, acting like a Trojan horse to deliver the gene that coded for the SARS-CoV-2 spike protein, much like the mRNA vaccines.

In October 2022, the third type of COVID-19 vaccine became available in the United States. This vaccine, produced by Novavax, was made in a more traditional manner. Like the hepatitis B and HPV vaccines, the Novavax vaccine contains the purified SARS-CoV-2 spike protein plus an adjuvant.

DID YOU KNOW?

The COVID-19 vaccines were the fastest vaccines ever made. The SARS-CoV-2 virus was isolated and its genome sequenced by January 2020. Eleven months later, two large clinical trials involving more than seventy thousand participants were completed. Previously, the fastest vaccine ever made was the mumps vaccine, which took four years to make from virus isolation to commercial product.

THINGS TO DO

Watch these animations that show how the mRNA and adeno-virus vaccines work:

- "How COVID-19 mRNA Vaccines Work": https://www.youtube.com/watch?v=8nD6Q9XoSFw
- "How COVID-19 Viral Vector Vaccines Work": https://www.youtube.com/watch?v=2NDc9Q_m-Wo

Source: Vaccine Makers Project (VaccineMakers.org), Vaccine Education Center at Children's Hospital of Philadelphia. These and other science-based animations can be found on the Vaccine Makers Project YouTube channel: https://www.youtube.com/c/VaccineMakersProject.

Who Should Get the COVID-19 Vaccine?

The COVID-19 vaccine is recommended for everyone six months of age or older.

Who Should Avoid or Delay Getting the COVID-19 Vaccine?

Infants younger than six months of age and those who have had a severe allergic reaction to a previous dose of COVID-19 vaccine or one of its ingredients should not be vaccinated.

People with a precaution for COVID-19 vaccine should discuss the relative risks and benefits of vaccination with their health care provider to make an informed decision. People with precautions currently include:

- Those who have had a nonsevere allergic reaction to a previous dose (which occurred within four hours of vaccination) or who have a nonsevere allergy to a vaccine ingredient
- Those with moderate or severe illness (regardless of fever)
- Children and adults with a history of multisystem inflammatory syndrome; for children, this is known as MIS-C, and for adults, this is known as MIS-A

- Those who developed myocarditis or pericarditis (inflammation of the heart muscle or surrounding tissue) within three weeks of a previous dose

People who are severely immune compromised are unlikely to respond adequately to the vaccine, but they are still generally recommended to be vaccinated. It is important for people in this group to take an antiviral medicine, like Paxlovid or remdesivir, early in the course of the illness if they are infected.

> **DID YOU KNOW?**
>
> Although children younger than six months of age cannot receive COVID-19 vaccines, when a pregnant person is vaccinated, the unborn child gets antibodies through the placenta, protecting them in the first six months of life before they can be vaccinated themselves.

Does the COVID-19 Vaccine Work?

When the first two COVID-19 vaccines became available in December 2020, they were shown to be about 95 percent effective at preventing mild, moderate, and severe disease. Six months after vaccines were available, protection against severe disease remained high, but protection against mild illness decreased to about 50 percent.

The goal of all COVID-19 vaccines is to prevent severe illness for as long as possible. Like other respiratory viruses, such as influenza, protection against mild disease won't last for very long.

The good news is that for otherwise healthy people younger than sixty-five years of age, protection against severe illness, afforded by either three doses of an mRNA vaccine (with the third dose administered at least four months after the second dose) or two doses plus a natural infection, appears to last for a long time. At least as far as we know now.

What Are the Side Effects of the COVID-19 Vaccine?

Like all vaccines, the COVID-19 vaccines can cause pain or redness as the injection site. It can also cause side effects associated with a vigorous immune response, such as low-grade fever, headache, muscle aches, joint aches, and fatigue, which can last for a few days.

One serious side effect of COVID-19 vaccines, particularly the mRNA versions, is myocarditis, an inflammation of the heart muscle. Myocarditis has also occurred rarely following vaccination with the Novavax purified-protein vaccine. Fortunately, this side effect appears to be short-lived and self-resolving. Although this side effect can occur in anyone after any dose, it most often occurs in boys and young men within a week of the second dose. The overall incidence of this side effect is about one in fifty thousand vaccine recipients, but in boys sixteen and seventeen years of age, myocarditis following vaccination can be as common as one in 6,600. In children between five and thirteen years of age, it occurs in about one in five hundred thousand vaccine recipients. Importantly, myocarditis is also caused by infection with SARS-CoV-2 virus, where it occurs more frequently than following vaccination and is often more severe. For this reason, choosing not to get the COVID-19 vaccine because of concerns about myocarditis does not actually reduce a person's risk of experiencing this condition.

The Janssen/J&J vaccine has been found to cause two severe side effects: thrombosis with thrombocytopenia syndrome (TTS) and Guillain-Barré syndrome (GBS). TTS is a condition characterized by simultaneous increase in blood clots and decrease in platelets, the cells responsible for blood clotting. As a result of these two severe side effects, this type of COVID-19 vaccine was recommended only for use in very limited situations and was subsequently removed from the market in the United States. Most people in the United States received mRNA-based COVID-19 vaccines. The Janssen/J&J vaccine is no longer available in the United States.

DID YOU KNOW?

COVID-19 can cause a postinfectious inflammatory disease in children called multisystem inflammatory syndrome in children (MIS-C). In typical cases, children have a mild or asymptomatic infection that resolves completely. Then, about one month later, they come to the hospital with a high fever and a combination of lung, liver, kidney, or heart disease. About 75 of 100 children with MIS-C have myocarditis. As of the beginning of 2023, about nine thousand children, usually between five and thirteen years of age, had been hospitalized with MIS-C, and about seventy had died. Adults can also experience this syndrome in what is known as MIS-A.

DID YOU KNOW?

Although myocarditis can occur after vaccination, myocarditis following a natural COVID-19 infection (with or without MIS-C or MIS-A) is more common and more severe.

Why Get the COVID-19 Vaccine?

Although the COVID-19 pandemic has subsided, SARS-CoV-2 virus continues to circulate and cause disease. It will likely circulate for decades to come, now joining the pantheon of winter respiratory viruses, like influenza and RSV, and contributing to the hundreds of thousands of hospitalizations and tens of thousands of deaths caused by respiratory viruses every year. Those most likely to benefit from a yearly COVID-19 vaccine are those most likely to be hospitalized or die if infected, such as older people, those with high-risk medical conditions, those who are immune compromised, and pregnant people.

Previously unvaccinated people trying to decide whether to vaccinate themselves or their unvaccinated, healthy children should consider the following:

1. *Anyone can die from COVID-19.* By February 2024, almost 1.2 million people in the United States had died from COVID-19; almost 1,800 of them were children.

2. *Even mild disease can lead to complications.* Children between five and thirteen years of age are the group most likely to suffer from MIS-C, and those younger than thirteen years of age are unlikely to suffer the most severe side effect of vaccination, myocarditis. As such, vaccinating children as soon as they are eligible offers the best opportunity to provide protection against a disease that they will be exposed to every winter.

3. *Each year's birth cohort offers a new group of people susceptible to infection.* Each year, three to four million children are born in the United States who, by the time they are six months old, will be fully susceptible to COVID-19.

4. *Questions remain about long COVID.* We are still learning about the lingering effects of COVID-19. The more severe an individual's infection, the more likely they are to suffer long-term effects. Vaccination has been shown to decrease severe disease and development of long COVID.

5. *The vaccines are safe.* mRNA vaccines, which are highly effective at preventing severe disease, have now been given safely to hundreds of millions of people, including tens of millions of children.

Vaccination affords the best chance to protect oneself and one's family against hospitalization or death from COVID-19. For these reasons, the choice of whether to get the COVID-19 vaccine should be an easy one.

COVID-19: OTHER THINGS YOU MIGHT HAVE WONDERED ABOUT

Long COVID

Some children and adults experience long-lasting symptoms after the initial COVID-19 infection has resolved. This has been termed long COVID and includes symptoms such as fatigue, lethargy, and "brain fog." The cause or causes of long COVID are still poorly understood. But those who are vaccinated have less of a chance of experiencing this condition.

Will We Need Annual COVID-19 Vaccinations?

Some people might need to get a yearly vaccine. It is incumbent upon the CDC to determine who is being hospitalized and who is dying from COVID-19 now that the pandemic has subsided. How old are they? What other medical conditions do they have? Have they been vaccinated? If so, what vaccine did they receive, and when did they last get it? Did they take antiviral drugs? Once this information is in hand, it will be clearer which groups are most likely to benefit from yearly vaccination. However, early evidence suggests that four groups are most likely to benefit from annual vaccination against COVID-19: adults sixty-five years and older; those with chronic conditions that increase their risk for severe disease, including chronic heart, lung, kidney, or liver disease; those who are immune compromised because of illness or medical treatment; and pregnant people.

COVID-19 and Animals

SARS-CoV-2 can affect more than three dozen different mammals, including common pets, like dogs and cats; livestock and zoo animals, particularly mink, big cats, nonhuman primates, manatees, and hippos; and wild animals, including white-tailed and mule deer. While animals have been demonstrated to be infected by people, few cases of animals transmitting the virus to people have been documented. Most often, these cases followed close contact between an individual and an infected animal.

COVID-19: Additional Resources

ONLINE INFORMATION

"COVID-19": https://www.cdc.gov/coronavirus/2019-nCoV/index .html

COVID-19: https://www.vaccineinformation.org/diseases/covid-19/

"COVID-19: The Disease vs the Vaccine": https://media.chop.edu
/data/files/pdfs/vec-covid-vs-vaccine-infographic.pdf

"COVID-19 Vaccines": https://www.voicesforvaccines.org/vaccine
-information/covid19/

"COVID-19 Vaccines: What You Should Know": https://media.chop
.edu/data/files/pdfs/vaccine-education-center-covid-qa.pdf

"A Look at Each Vaccine: COVID-19 Vaccine": https://www.chop.edu
/centers-programs/vaccine-education-center/vaccine-details/covid
-19-vaccine

"My COVID-19 Vaccine Experience": https://www.chop.edu/centers
-programs/vaccine-education-center/resources/vaccine-videos
-and-dvds/covid19-vaccine-experience

"Perspectives on COVID-19 Vaccine for Kids": https://www.chop.edu
/centers-programs/vaccine-education-center/resources/vaccine
-videos-and-dvds/perspectives-covid-19-vaccine-kids

"Questions and Answers About COVID-19 Vaccines": COVIDVac-
cineAnswers.org

"Rare, but Severe, Side Effects Following COVID-19 Vaccination":
https://media.chop.edu/data/files/pdfs/side-effects-covid-19
-infographic.pdf

"Talking About Vaccines with Dr. Hank Bernstein: COVID-19": https://
www.chop.edu/centers-programs/vaccine-education-center
/resources/vaccine-videos-and-dvds/talking-about-vaccines
-hank-bernstein

"Talking About Vaccines with Dr. Paul Offit: COVID-19": https://
www.chop.edu/centers-programs/vaccine-education-center
/resources/vaccine-videos-and-dvds/covid-19

PERSONAL EXPERIENCES

"Story Gallery": https://www.shotbyshot.org/story-gallery/ (search
"COVID-19")

SUPPORT GROUPS

Long COVID Support was started by a group of people "struggling
to recover from COVID-19." They offer support, advocacy, and
research participation opportunities: https://www.longcovid.org.

BOOKS

Lewis, Michael. *The Premonition: A Pandemic Story.* New York: W. W. Norton, 2021.

Offit, Paul A., *Tell Me When It's Over: An Insider's Guide to Deciphering COVID Myths and Navigating Our Post-Pandemic World.* Washington, DC: National Geographic, 2024.

VACCINES IN THE SECOND YEAR OF LIFE

During the second year of life, babies get two distinct groups of vaccines. One is additional doses of vaccines they had in the first few months of life. Except for influenza vaccine, giving additional doses several months after the most recent dose in the first year of life builds stronger immunologic memory. As with all other age groups influenza vaccine is recommended in the second year of life because of how quickly the virus changes, often nullifying immunity gained in the previous season.

The second group of vaccines given in the second year of life are new. These include measles-mumps-rubella (MMR), chickenpox (varicella), and hepatitis A vaccines.

VACCINES TO REVISIT

DTaP Vaccine

Children are recommended to get a fourth dose of the diphtheria, tetanus, and pertussis vaccine known as DTaP between fifteen and eighteen months of age. See the "Diphtheria, Tetanus, and Pertussis" section of the "Vaccines in the First Year of Life" chapter for details about these diseases and the DTaP vaccine.

Hib Vaccine

Depending which brand of *Haemophilus influenzae* type b (Hib) vaccine a child received as an infant, they are recommended to get a third or fourth dose between twelve and fifteen months of age. See the "*Haemophilus Influenzae* Type b (Hib)" section of the "Vaccines in the First Year of Life" chapter for details about this disease and the Hib vaccine.

Pneumococcal Vaccine

Children are recommended to get a fourth dose of pneumococcal vaccine between twelve and fifteen months of age. They should receive the same version they got for the first three doses whenever possible (PCV15 or PCV20). For more information about pneumococcus and the vaccines to prevent it, see the "Pneumococcus" section of the "Vaccines in the First Year of Life" chapter.

Influenza Vaccine

Most children should have received two doses of influenza vaccine separated by a month during the first year of life. However, depending on the time of year they were born relative to influenza season, they may have received no doses or just one dose. If the child did not receive two doses in the first year of life, they will need two doses separated by four weeks during the second year of life. To get more details about influenza and the vaccine, check the "Influenza" section of the "Vaccines in the First Year of Life" chapter.

MEASLES, MUMPS, AND RUBELLA (MMR)

MEASLES, MUMPS, AND RUBELLA: THE DISEASES

Since a fraudulent report suggested that the MMR vaccine could cause autism, parents have wondered about its safety. After this hypothesis was put forth, several studies conducted on multiple continents by numerous independent groups of scientists analyzed data from hundreds of thousands of children—no study found evidence linking the MMR vaccine with autism. Unfortunately, many parents today continue to be exposed to misinformation suggesting something where there is nothing. Sadly, some of those parents act on this ill-founded guidance, leaving their children vulnerable to dangerous diseases while not changing their risk of autism by one iota.

The MMR vaccine protects against three troublesome viruses: measles, mumps, and rubella. Each disease spreads quickly, can cause severe complications, and sometimes results in death. Even a small drop in vaccination rates can lead to outbreaks.

Between 2014 and 2015, a measles outbreak stemming from a community in Southern California near Disneyland led to more than one hundred cases being diagnosed across seven states and two other countries (Canada and Mexico). In 2018, outbreaks in three states led to 375 cases. More worrisome were cases in 2019, which numbered almost 1,300 and were detected in thirty-one states. At the end of December 2022, schools and day care centers in Columbus, Ohio, reported eighty-five cases of measles in children, 70 percent of which occurred in those less than two years of age. Thirty-two children were hospitalized. In each outbreak, almost all those infected had not been immunized.

Between 2015 and 2019, almost twenty thousand people were diagnosed with mumps. About 9,200 of these cases occurred as a result of 150 outbreaks between January 2016 and June 2017. The outbreaks occurred in households, workplaces, schools and colleges, on athletic teams, at churches, and following large parties or events. In the first nine months of 2023, more than three hundred cases of mumps were reported in thirty-nine states.

All of this suffering was entirely preventable.

What Is Measles?

Measles is a virus spread from one person to another by small droplets that hang in the air. Measles virus is quite contagious; indeed, if one hundred susceptible people are in a room with someone who has measles, about ninety will get the disease.

Those at highest risk of measles include college students, international travelers, and health care providers.

> **DID YOU KNOW?**
>
> People can be infected by measles virus that remains in the air up to two hours after a person with measles has left the area.

What Are the Symptoms of Measles?

Measles occurs most often in late winter and spring. People with measles typically experience:

- Fever that gradually increases, reaching between 103°F and 105°F
- Cough, runny nose, and conjunctivitis (pink eye)
- Raised, bluish-white spots on the inside of the mouth (called Koplik spots, they are a defining characteristic of this disease)
- Rash consisting of red spots that are raised in the middle. The rash usually begins around the hairline, moves to the face and upper neck, and gradually spreads downward and outward until it reaches the hands and feet. The rash tends to fade in the same order that it appeared
- Diarrhea and lack of appetite, most commonly occurring in infants

About 30 of 100 people with measles will experience complications, most often children younger than five years of age and adults older than nineteen years of age. Complications can include:

- Ear infection occurs in about seven of 100 people.
- Diarrhea occurs in about eight of 100 people; in resource-limited settings, the dehydration caused by diarrhea can be fatal.
- Pneumonia occurs in about six of 100 people; this complication is the most common cause of death, particularly in children. Pneumonia is caused by either the measles virus itself or bacteria (like pneumococcus) that take advantage of an immune system weakened by measles.

- Encephalitis (brain inflammation) occurs in about one of 1,000 people and causes fever, headache, vomiting, stiff neck, drowsiness, seizures, and occasionally coma. About 15 of 100 people with this complication die. Of those who survive, about 25 of 100 will suffer permanent brain damage. Adults who die from measles most commonly experience this complication.
- Death occurs in about one of five hundred people. Before measles vaccine was introduced in the United States in 1963, the virus killed five hundred to one thousand people every year, most were previously healthy children.
- Subacute sclerosing panencephalitis (SSPE), a rare progressive, unrelenting neurological disorder suffered by people who have recovered from measles. SSPE causes mental deterioration, loss of muscle control, seizures, and muscle twitching. It occurs in about 100 to 400 of every million people, and it is devastating, invariably causing death. SSPE has occurred as soon as one month and as long as twenty-seven years after infection, but generally it occurs between five and ten years after the infection. SSPE has virtually disappeared since introduction of the measles vaccine.
- Hemorrhagic measles is a rare complication causing high fever (105–106°F), seizures, difficulty breathing, bleeding under the skin, and delirium.
- Clotting disorder caused by a low platelet count (platelets are cells in the bloodstream that help the blood to clot) can also be a rare complication of measles.

ONE PERSON'S STORY

Recalling his experience treating measles, a retired pediatrician who practiced in Alaska wrote, "One day I was on the neurological ward at the Children's Hospital and saw a very handsome lad of about ten years old. He was sitting in a large crib and rocking back and forth, staring vacantly, and moaning. When

I reviewed his chart, it revealed that he'd suffered the measles complication of encephalitis. This is unusual—one in a thousand cases incidence—but for this boy it meant he was left in a nonverbal, blind state from damage to his nervous system from the measles virus."

Source: Moss, Kenneth. "Unprotected People #29: Measles." Immunize. org. Accessed May 7, 2023. https://www.immunize.org/wp-content /uploads/reports/report029.pdf.

Measles infections can be particularly damaging in pregnant people and people who are immune compromised. Pregnant people who get measles are more likely to deliver early, have miscarriages, or deliver babies with low birth weight. Although people who are immune compromised do not always have a rash when infected with measles, the disease tends to be more severe and longer-lasting in them than in otherwise healthy people.

THINGS TO DO

Because of the danger of measles infection during pregnancy, people considering pregnancy should make sure they are immune to measles before conceiving.

What Is Mumps?

Mumps is caused by a virus that spreads from one person to another by coughing, sneezing, or contact with the saliva of an infected person. Mumps is not as contagious as measles, but it's still spread easily. Adults at increased risk include health care workers, international travelers, and college students. As is true for measles and chickenpox, adults with mumps are usually more severely ill than children.

DID YOU KNOW?

To determine how easily a disease spreads, public health officials measure how many susceptible people become ill when they have been exposed to the disease. Mumps is less contagious than measles and chickenpox but about as contagious as influenza and rubella.

What Are the Symptoms of Mumps?

People with mumps can have:

- No symptoms occur in about 20 of 100 people.
- Nonspecific symptoms occur in about 45 of 100 people and include body aches, lack of appetite, headache, and low-grade fever.
- Swollen glands occur in about 97 of 100 people and last for about ten days. In addition to the nonspecific symptoms mentioned above, some people have swollen parotid glands, which are located at the angle of the jaw below the ear and help to digest food. Swelling of these glands makes children look like chipmunks. The swelling can lead to earaches and tenderness in the jaw.

Although symptoms of mumps aren't severe, complications can be devastating and may include:

- Meningitis (inflammation of the lining of the brain and spinal cord) occurs in about five of 100 people. Before the mumps vaccine was first used in the United States in the mid-1960s, mumps was the most common cause of viral meningitis.
- Encephalitis (inflammation of the brain) occurs in about two of 100,000 people.
- Orchitis (swelling and tenderness of the testicle) occurs in about 30 of 100 postpubertal males. Other symptoms include nausea, vomiting, and fever.
- Oophoritis (inflammation of the ovary) occurs in about five of 100 postpubertal females. Fortunately, oophoritis does not appear to affect fertility.

- Mastitis (inflammation of the mammary gland) occurs in about 30 of 100 postpubertal females.
- Pancreatitis (inflammation of the pancreas) occurs in about four of 100 people. Pancreatitis can occur soon after infection, causing severe abdominal pain, nausea, and fever.
- Deafness occurs in about four of 100 people.
- Myocarditis (inflammation of the heart) occurs in about nine of 100 people and in most cases resolves without incident. Rarely, however, myocarditis can be fatal.
- Miscarriage has been suggested by some studies as a potential complication of mumps infection during the first trimester of pregnancy; however, not all studies have shown this.

THINGS TO DO

Because of the theoretical increased risk of miscarriage, people considering pregnancy should make sure they are immune to mumps before conceiving.

What Is Rubella?

Rubella, also called German measles, is a virus that spreads from person to person by coughing, sneezing, or exposure to the saliva of an infected person. Rubella virus causes two distinct illnesses: rubella and congenital rubella syndrome.

What Are the Symptoms of Rubella?

People with rubella may experience:

- No symptoms occur in about half those infected with rubella.
- Symptoms of mild disease typically include fever, swollen glands, and a rash that first appears on the face and neck and then spreads downward. Some people also develop conjunctivitis (pink eye). Adults, particularly women, also commonly experience short-lived arthritis (joint swelling and pain).

• Disease with complications is more likely to occur in adults than in children; complications include encephalitis (swelling of the brain; occurs in about one of six thousand people, more often in females) and thrombocytopenia (low platelet count; occurs in about one of 3,000 people and although scary, is typically short-lived).

Congenital rubella syndrome (CRS) is the most devastating outcome of rubella infection and is the main reason that people are immunized. Unborn babies are most likely to develop CRS if their mother is infected before the twentieth week of gestation; in fact, up to 85 of 100 babies will be affected if infection occurs during the first trimester.

CRS can cause fetal death, miscarriage, or premature delivery. In addition, developing fetuses who survive often suffer permanent damage that can include:

• Deafness (the most common outcome)
• Cataracts, glaucoma, or other eye damage
• Heart murmur or other heart damage
• Lack of head growth
• Cognitive developmental delay
• Skeletal damage
• Liver or spleen damage
• Diabetes
• Autism

DID YOU KNOW?

The irony of the unfounded fear that MMR vaccine causes autism is that the vaccine actually *prevents* a small number of children from getting autism by preventing CRS.

MMR: THE VACCINE

What Is the MMR Vaccine?

The MMR vaccine is three vaccines in one. Each is made from live, weakened versions of the viruses (see "How Are Vaccines Made?").

Measles vaccine. The weakened version of measles virus in the vaccine is called the Moraten strain, and it has been used to protect against measles since 1968. This strain is "more attenuated" (hence, "Moraten") than a previous measles vaccine.

> **DID YOU KNOW?**
>
> A few other measles vaccines were used before 1968 but caused more side effects. An inactivated vaccine was used between 1963 and 1967; however, it didn't work particularly well, and people who got measles after getting that vaccine suffered "atypical measles," which caused fever, pneumonia, and an unusual rash, often appearing first on the wrists or ankles. For this reason, the inactivated vaccine was removed from the market.

Mumps vaccine. The weakened version of mumps virus used in the MMR vaccine is known as the Jeryl Lynn strain; it was first available in 1967. The vaccine is named for the five-year-old girl from whom the virus was isolated, Jeryl Lynn Hilleman. Dr. Maurice Hilleman, her father, was a scientist working at Merck Sharpe and Dohme. When Jeryl Lynn got mumps, he swabbed her throat, took the virus to the lab, weakened it, and used it as the vaccine.

> **DID YOU KNOW?**
>
> Dr. Hilleman is credited with saving millions of lives by developing more than half the vaccines routinely given to infants and
>
> (*continued on next page*)

(continued from previous page)

young children. Yet many people have never heard of him. To learn more about the Jeryl Lynn story and all of Dr. Hilleman's accomplishments, check out the book *Vaccinated: One Man's Quest to Defeat the World's Deadliest Diseases* (New York: Smithsonian Books, 2007) or the award-winning documentary, *Hilleman: A Perilous Quest to Save the World's Children* (Medical History Pictures, Inc., 2016), available at https://hillemanfilm.com/.

DID YOU KNOW?

Dr. Stanley Plotkin, the inventor of the rubella vaccine, is sometimes accused of making an unethical decision when he opted to grow the rubella vaccine virus in fetal cells. However, at the time, he was racing against the clock to protect mothers and their unborn babies from an impending rubella epidemic, and scientists had recently determined that some animal cell lines were contaminated with other viruses. Dr. Plotkin discussed his experience and how this led to his choice in the documentary *Stanley Plotkin: Pioneering the Use of Fetal Cells to Make Rubella Vaccine* (Medical History Pictures, 2019), available at https://hillemanfilm.com/stanley-plotkin.

Rubella vaccine. The weakened version of rubella virus used in the MMR vaccine became available in 1979. The virus was originally isolated in Philadelphia in 1965 from a fetus who died of rubella. Whereas the measles and mumps vaccine viruses are both weakened by growth in chick embryo cells, the rubella vaccine virus is weakened by adaptation to growth at lower temperatures in human embryo cells (see "How Are Vaccines Made?" and "Are Vaccines Made Using Aborted Fetal Cells?").

Who Should Get the MMR Vaccine?

The MMR vaccine is recommended as a series of two shots for all children: one between twelve and fifteen months of age and the other between four and six years of age. The vaccine is delayed until at least twelve months because maternal antibodies passed through the placenta can interfere with an infant's immune response in the first year of life.

DID YOU KNOW?

Adults born before 1957 are considered to be immune to measles, mumps, and rubella because those infections were so common then. However, if someone born before 1957 works in a health care field and does not have proof of infection or vaccination, they are recommended to get one or two doses of MMR vaccine, depending on which disease they do not have evidence of protection against.

THINGS TO DO

Because measles, mumps, and rubella occur more commonly in other parts of the world, international travelers should be sure they are immune before traveling.

Does the MMR Vaccine Work?

Of every hundred children who have received the first dose of MMR, ninety-six will be protected against measles, eighty-three against mumps, and ninety against rubella. The second dose of the vaccine provides increased protection against all three viruses.

Who Should Avoid or Delay Getting the MMR Vaccine?

Pregnant people, people who are immune compromised, and those who have had a severe allergic reaction to a previous dose or to a vaccine ingredient should not get MMR vaccine. However, people considering pregnancy can be reassured by the fact that hundreds of pregnant people have inadvertently been given MMR without damage to their unborn children. The risks to the unborn child are theoretical only.

People who are moderately or severely ill, those who recently received blood products, people with a blood-clotting condition, and those requiring tuberculin skin testing or interferon-gamma release assay testing should delay getting the vaccine.

What Are the Side Effects of MMR Vaccine?

MMR vaccine is generally safe but can cause some mild side effects, including:

- Fever occurs in about 10 of 100 people and is typically caused by the measles component of the vaccine or, rarely, by the rubella component.
- Rash occurs in about five of 100 people within a week to ten days of receiving the vaccine and is typically caused by the measles component.
- Arthritis or joint inflammation occurs rarely in children but can occur in as many as 25 of 100 adults who get the vaccine, mostly women; this side effect is typically associated with the rubella component and usually goes away within three weeks.
- Thrombocytopenia (low platelet count) occurs in about one of 25,000 people up to six weeks after getting the vaccine. This disorder doesn't usually cause any problems and goes away on its own.
- Seizures associated with fever occur in about one of three thousand to four thousand children and are attributed to the measles component.

Why Get the MMR Vaccine?

1. *Measles and mumps continue to occur in the United States.* Outbreaks of both continue to occur each year.

2. *Rubella can be devastating to a developing fetus.* While a child may not experience complications from rubella, the unborn babies of people who are infected during pregnancy can be killed or permanently harmed.

3. *Measles complications are common in young children and adults.* Children less than five years old are most likely to experience complications, including ear infections and pneumonia. Adults are also more likely to experience severe disease and complications.

4. *Although rare, measles infections can cause the invariably fatal disease SSPE.* Unlike measles infections, the measles vaccine does not cause SSPE.

5. *Mumps can cause deafness.* Hundreds to thousands of cases of mumps continue to occur in the United States every year.

6. *Measles, mumps, and rubella can all be harmful to pregnant people.* Because immunity is lifelong, immunization in childhood will protect future mothers.

7. *The vaccine is safe.* Although side effects occur, they are mild.

MMR: OTHER THINGS YOU MIGHT HAVE WONDERED ABOUT
MMR and Autism

The MMR vaccine does not cause autism. To read more about the science and history of this concern, see "Do Vaccines Cause Autism?"

Individual Vaccines

Some parents prefer to give MMR as three separate vaccines, believing this makes the vaccines safer (see "Do Vaccines Cause Autism?" and "Can Too Many Vaccines Weaken the Immune System?"). However, separating these vaccines does not make them safer; rather, it only prolongs the interval during which children are susceptible to the diseases. It also means more shots and more doctor visits. Currently, these three vaccines are not available separately in the United States.

Boys and the Rubella Vaccine

Because rubella is most dangerous when it infects pregnant people, some might wonder why we immunize boys and men. In fact, we immunize them for three reasons. First, boys can get sick from rubella and on rare occasions experience complications of the infection, such as encephalitis. Second, immunizing the entire population means that rubella virus has less opportunity to circulate in the community and cause disease. Third, decreasing the chance that boys and men are infected with rubella protects any pregnant people that they are near.

MMR: Additional Resources

ONLINE INFORMATION

"A Look at Each Vaccine: Measles, Mumps and Rubella (MMR) Vaccine": https://www.chop.edu/centers-programs/vaccine-education-center/vaccine-details/measles-mumps-and-rubella-vaccines

"Measles, Mumps, and Rubella (MMR) Vaccine": https://www.voicesforvaccines.org/vaccine-information/mmr/

"MMR": https://media.chop.edu/data/files/pdfs/mmr-infographic.pdf

"Doctors Talk: Measles": https://www.chop.edu/centers-programs/vaccine-education-center/video/doctors-talk-measles

"Measles": https://www.vaccineinformation.org/diseases/measles/

"Measles: What You Should Know": https://media.chop.edu/data/files/pdfs/vaccine-education-center-measles.pdf

"Hilleman – Mumps Segment – Vaccine Makers Project": https://www.youtube.com/watch?v=mQghyCeocP4

"Mumps": https://www.vaccineinformation.org/diseases/mumps/

"Mumps: What You Should Know": https://media.chop.edu/data/files/pdfs/vaccine-education-center-mumps.pdf

"Rubella": https://www.vaccineinformation.org/diseases/rubella/

"Vaccines and Autism: What You Should Know": https://media.chop.edu/data/files/pdfs/vaccine-education-center-autism.pdf

PHOTOS

"Measles Photos": https://www.vaccineinformation.org/photos/measles/
"Mumps Photos": https://www.vaccineinformation.org/photos/mumps/
"Rubella Photos": https://www.vaccineinformation.org/photos/rubella/

PERSONAL EXPERIENCES

"Parents PACK Personal Stories – Measles": https://www.chop.edu
/centers-programs/parents-pack/personal-stories/measles
"Story Gallery": https://www.shotbyshot.org/story-gallery/ (search
"measles" and "rubella")
"Unprotected People Stories: Measles": https://www.immunize.org
/clinical/vaccine-confidence/unprotected-people/topic/measles/
"Unprotected People Stories: Mumps": https://www.immunize.org
/clinical/vaccine-confidence/unprotected-people/topic/mumps/
"Unprotected People Stories: Rubella": https://www.immunize.org/clinical
/vaccine-confidence/unprotected-people/topic/rubella/

CHICKENPOX

CHICKENPOX: THE DISEASE

Chickenpox is an infection often thought of as a childhood rite of passage because before the vaccine, almost every child got the disease by the end of elementary school. Most parents remember the itchy rash, mild fever, and oatmeal baths that typically accompany chickenpox.

What Is Chickenpox?

Also known as varicella, chickenpox virus is highly contagious, passed from one person to another through small droplets that can hang in the air for hours. Indeed, about 90 of 100 people who have not had chickenpox will get the disease when exposed to someone who is infected.

What Are the Symptoms of Chickenpox?

Most children with chickenpox have:

- Fever of up to 102°F, lasting two to three days
- Rash composed of blisters that usually start on the head and spread to the rest of the body; typically, three hundred to five hundred blisters erupt
- Itching

Before the vaccine was first introduced in the United States in 1995, about ten thousand children were hospitalized and seventy killed by chickenpox every year. Hospitalizations and deaths were caused by:

- Severe infections of the skin caused by bacteria such as *staphylococcus* and *streptococcus*, specifically, necrotizing fasciitis (when bacteria rapidly spread through muscles) and pyomyositis (when bacteria cause pus to collect within muscles)
- Pneumonia

- Meningitis
- Encephalitis (inflammation of the brain) leading to seizures or coma

Even more rarely, people with chickenpox can develop Guillain-Barré syndrome (GBS), low platelet count, hemorrhage, arthritis, or inflammation of the heart, kidneys, testes, liver, or irises.

ONE PERSON'S STORY

"It was just a normal breakout of chickenpox, and one got severely infected under his arm. But it was just that one chickenpox. That's all it took. It turned into a flesh-eating disease. It was just a clear hole. You could see straight to the muscle, which we had to keep bandaged. He was very sick. He could have lost his arm. He could have died. It could have been really bad."

Source: Pugh, Carol. "Vaccines and Your Baby." Vaccine Education Center at Children's Hospital of Philadelphia. Last reviewed July 23, 2014. https://www.chop.edu/centers-programs/vaccine-education-center /video/vaccines-and-your-baby.

DID YOU KNOW?

Adults are more likely than children to die from chickenpox. About five of 100 cases of chickenpox occur in adults, but 35 of 100 who die from chickenpox are adults.

CHICKENPOX: THE VACCINE

What Is the Chickenpox Vaccine?

The chickenpox vaccine is made from live, weakened varicella virus. The virus used in the vaccine was originally taken from an otherwise healthy little boy with chickenpox in Japan in the 1970s. Once the virus was in the lab, it was grown in several other kinds of cells so that it would no longer grow well in people (see "How Are Vaccines Made?"). Now, when the virus is given to children as a vaccine, it can't grow well enough to make children ill, but it can grow well enough to induce a protective immune response.

DID YOU KNOW?

Like other viruses, chickenpox virus must reproduce inside cells. So, although researchers used a virus from a boy in Japan, they had to use cells isolated from another source to grow it. The cells used to make the chickenpox vaccine are human cells obtained from an elective termination of a pregnancy in the early 1960s. These cells continue to grow in the laboratory. Human cells are used to make not only the chickenpox vaccine but also the rubella and hepatitis A vaccines, as well as one version of the rabies vaccine and one version of the COVID-19 vaccine (see "Are Vaccines Made Using Aborted Fetal Cells?").

Who Should Get the Chickenpox Vaccine?

Two doses of the chickenpox vaccine are recommended for all children who have not previously had chickenpox documented by a health care professional or laboratory test result. The first dose should be received between twelve and fifteen months of age and the second between four and six years of age. Children older than six years of age and adults born after 1980 who have not received two doses of this vaccine should also be vaccinated. The timing between doses depends on the age of the individual being vaccinated.

Although adults born before 1980 are likely to have immunity against varicella, two groups should not rely on their birth year alone to assume immunity. First, people who work in health care must have proof of immunity in the form of vaccination, documented infection, or a laboratory test. Because they are at higher risk for exposure, they should have two doses of vaccine if they do not have proof of immunity. Second, because a chickenpox infection during pregnancy can harm the fetus, immunity should be confirmed before conceiving. If lack of immunity is not discovered until a person is pregnant, vaccine doses should be administered after delivery.

THINGS TO DO

Adults who have not had chickenpox or the chickenpox vaccine are at greater risk of experiencing severe disease and complications if infected; therefore, they should get two doses of the vaccine separated by at least one month.

Does the Chickenpox Vaccine Work?

After one dose of chickenpox vaccine, about 80 of 100 children will be protected against moderate and severe disease; however, about 20 of 100 may have a mild case, known as breakthrough disease, if they are exposed to chickenpox. The second dose of vaccine helps to protect the children who were not fully protected after the first dose. After two doses, about 90 of 100 children are protected against even mild disease.

Who Should Delay or Avoid Getting the Chickenpox Vaccine?

The following individuals have a "precaution" for chickenpox vaccine, meaning they should delay getting the chickenpox vaccine or discuss the relative risks and benefits of vaccination with their health care provider:

- Those with moderate or severe illnesses (excluding mild fever, ear infection, mild respiratory infection, or mild diarrheal illness)

- Those who recently received antibody-containing blood products (e.g., immunoglobulin)
- Those taking certain antiviral medications in the twenty-four hours before vaccination
- Those using aspirin-containing products

The following groups should not get the chickenpox vaccine:

- Those with cancer (e.g., leukemia, lymphoma) and certain immunodeficiencies
- People receiving long-term immunosuppressive therapy (e.g., bone marrow or solid organ transplant recipients)
- Those receiving high doses of steroids by mouth (see "Can I Get Vaccinated If I'm Taking Steroids?")
- People who have had a severe allergic reaction to a previous dose of the vaccine or one of its ingredients, such as gelatin (see "Do Vaccines Cause Allergies or Asthma?")
- Those who are pregnant

Because these people need to be protected from exposure to chickenpox virus, it is important for those around them to be immune.

THINGS TO DO

If someone in your family cannot get chickenpox vaccine, you can minimize the risk of getting chickenpox by:

- Making sure everyone else in your household has already had chickenpox or been immunized
- Keeping the unvaccinated family member away from others who have chickenpox
- If a child, making sure the school nurse or other staff member is aware of the child's susceptibility to this illness

This is particularly important since people who cannot get chickenpox vaccine are most likely to suffer severe disease or complications.

ONE PERSON'S STORY

"Christopher was born a very healthy child, but at the age of eight he developed asthma. It was never a problem for him, and it never kept him from doing things he loved. But on June 16, 1988, four years after he was diagnosed, he suffered his first and only severe asthma attack. He had to be hospitalized and was treated with all of the normally prescribed drugs. . . . On June 23, exactly one week after the asthma attack, he broke out with the chickenpox. 'Don't worry, you'll get over it,' I told him. What I didn't know was that the corticosteroid [taken for asthma] had lowered his body's immune response and he could not fight the disease. The chickenpox began to rampage wildly through his young body. As I drove him to the emergency room on June 27, my four younger children watched silently in shock and horror as their brother went into seizures, went blind, turned gray, and collapsed due to hemorrhaging in his brain."

Source: Cole, Rebecca. "Chickenpox Claimed the Life of My Son Christopher." Immunize.org. November 16, 1999. https://www
.immunize.org/clinical/vaccine-confidence/unprotected-people
/story/chickenpox-claimed-the-life-of-my-son-christopher/#:~:text=
Christopher%20was%20born%20a%20very,and%20only%20severe%20
asthma%20attack.

What Are the Side Effects of the Chickenpox Vaccine?

The chickenpox vaccine may cause mild side effects:

- Minor pain, redness, or swelling at the injection site occurs in about 20 of 100 people
- Rash near the injection site occurs in about four of 100 people
- Rash distant from the injection site occurs in about four of 100 people

DID YOU KNOW?

Rashes occurring after receipt of chickenpox vaccine may have as few as three to five blisters, far fewer than the three hundred to five hundred that develop during a typical chickenpox infection.

Why Get the Chickenpox Vaccine?

1. *Chickenpox is still around.* The chickenpox vaccine became available in 1995. Every year before that, about four million people in the United States got chickenpox, and about one hundred died. The year 2020 marked twenty-five years of using this vaccine in the United States. As a result, each year there are fewer than 150,000 cases of chickenpox and fewer than thirty deaths. Although these numbers are much lower than before the vaccine was available, people are still getting sick and dying from chickenpox.
2. *Some people suffer complications from chickenpox, and some die.* Although most people experience a relatively minor case, some people are at higher risk of suffering severe disease or complications, and unfortunately, every year about thirty people still die from this disease in the United States.
3. *Some people can't get the chickenpox vaccine and need others to protect them.* Some people are unable to get the vaccine and must rely on those around them to be protected (see "Is It My Social Responsibility to Get Vaccinated?").
4. *The vaccine provides protection from shingles as an adult.* People who get the chickenpox vaccine are less likely to suffer from shingles (a painful rash that occurs when either the natural virus or the vaccine virus reactivates) later in life.
5. *The vaccine is safe.* Side effects are relatively rare and mild.

CHICKENPOX: OTHER THINGS YOU MIGHT
HAVE WONDERED ABOUT
Chickenpox Parties

Before the chickenpox vaccine became available in 1995, some parents intentionally exposed their children to the disease at "chickenpox parties." The purpose was to allow children to get sick at an age when they were less likely to experience severe illness, complications, or death from chickenpox. But now that a chickenpox vaccine is available, there's a safer way to protect children from severe disease and complications.

Unfortunately, chickenpox parties are still sometimes held. However, because of the success of the vaccine, it's not as easy to find someone with chickenpox, so some parents take out ads online, find information on message boards, have clothing from infected children mailed to them, or go to the homes of strangers. During chickenpox parties, children are encouraged to share lollipops, cups, and clothing to increase their chances of getting chickenpox naturally. These parties are an extreme and dangerous way to provide immunity, given the safety of the vaccine, the chance of suffering severe complications and death from natural disease, and the contrast with what we try to teach our children about avoiding other infections (e.g., covering their cough, not sharing food or drinks, not putting toys in their mouths).

Chickenpox in Older Children and Adults

People fifteen years of age and older are more likely to experience complications or die from chickenpox. If adolescents or adults have not had the chickenpox vaccine or been diagnosed with chickenpox by a doctor, they should get two doses of the vaccine. Although it's preferable to be immune to chickenpox before becoming pregnant, those who are pregnant should wait until after delivery to get immunized. The chickenpox vaccine can be given safely during the period of breastfeeding (see "Can I Get Vaccinated If I'm Pregnant or Breastfeeding?").

Immunizing Your Older Children While You're Pregnant

Children who recently received the chickenpox vaccine do not pose a threat to pregnant people; therefore, if you have children who need to be vaccinated, it is safe to immunize them while you are pregnant.

The Chickenpox Vaccine as a Cause of Shingles

The virus that causes chickenpox lives silently in a person's body after they've had a natural chickenpox infection or the chickenpox vaccine. Shingles occurs when either the natural virus or the vaccine virus reactivates to cause a painful rash. However, since the vaccine virus grows much less efficiently in people than the natural virus, the likelihood of getting shingles is lower and, if shingles does develop, the symptoms are milder and shorter-lived after vaccination than after natural infection.

How to Protect Your Baby if Grandma Has Shingles

Shingles typically occurs when a person has a weakened immune system due to age or disease. Because it is the reactivation of a virus that is already living in a person's body, one person cannot give another person shingles. However, a person with shingles can give chickenpox to someone who has never had chickenpox or the chickenpox vaccine. This can happen only if the non-immune person comes into contact with the rash before it has crusted. It is not typically transmitted by coughing, sneezing, or casual contact.

DID YOU KNOW?

Although babies do not receive the chickenpox vaccine until twelve months of age, very young infants are likely to be protected by antibodies transferred through the placenta before birth. It is because of these short-lived but protective antibodies that some viral vaccines, such as chickenpox and MMR vaccines, are not given until twelve months. Before then, maternal antibodies may interfere with development of the baby's own immune response.

THINGS TO DO

A shingles vaccine is now available for people fifty years of age and older. This two-dose vaccine provides a boost in immunity to decrease the chance of getting shingles (see the shingles section in the "Vaccines for Adults" chapter for more information.)

Chickenpox: Additional Resources

ONLINE INFORMATION

"Chickenpox (Varicella)": https://www.vaccineinformation.org/diseases /chickenpox/

"Chickenpox Vaccine": https://www.voicesforvaccines.org/vaccine -information/chickenpox/

"Chickenpox Vaccine Saves Lives and Prevents Serious Illness Info-graphic": https://www.cdc.gov/chickenpox/vaccine-infographic.html

"Chickenpox: What You Should Know": https://media.chop.edu/data /files/pdfs/vaccine-education-center-chickenpox.pdf

"A Look at Each Vaccine: Varicella Vaccine": https://www.chop.edu /centers-programs/vaccine-education-center/vaccine-details/varicella -vaccine

PHOTOS

"Chickenpox Photos": https://www.vaccineinformation.org/photos /chickenpox/

"Parents PACK Personal Stories – Chickenpox": https://www.chop .edu/centers-programs/parents-pack/personal-stories/chickenpox

"Story Gallery": https://www.shotbyshot.org/story-gallery/ (search "chickenpox")

"Unprotected People Stories: Varicella (Chickenpox)": https://www .immunize.org/clinical/vaccine-confidence/unprotected-people /topic/varicella-chickenpox/

HEPATITIS A

HEPATITIS A: THE DISEASE

Although you don't hear much about it, hepatitis A virus infects thousands of people in the United States every year. Between 2016 and the middle of 2023, about forty-five thousand cases of hepatitis A were reported in the United States, and more than twenty-seven thousand people had to be hospitalized. More than four hundred died. Two points are important here. First, these numbers are assumed to be low because officials know that many cases of hepatitis A go undetected. Second, these cases could have been prevented by vaccination.

While many cases of hepatitis A are associated with drug use, homelessness, and incarceration, each year, some cases result from everyday activities, like going to a restaurant, stopping at the local convenience store to pick up a quick meal, traveling internationally, or even consuming fresh vegetables or frozen fruit purchased from the local grocery store. The reality is that anyone can unwittingly be exposed to hepatitis A.

What Is Hepatitis A?

Hepatitis A is a virus spread by contaminated food and water. Symptoms typically occur about a month after exposure to the virus and last about two months. In about 10 of 100 people with hepatitis A, symptoms can last for six months.

Those at highest risk of hepatitis A infection include:

- International travelers to countries with high rates of hepatitis A, including parts of Africa and Asia, as well as Central and South America and Eastern Europe
- People who use drugs
- People experiencing homelessness or incarceration
- Men who have sex with men
- People with chronic liver disease

DID YOU KNOW?

Handwashing after changing diapers or using the restroom and before handling food can decrease the spread of hepatitis A virus. But handwashing isn't failproof. People are most likely to transmit the virus one to two weeks *before* their first symptoms appear, so many who are contagious don't know they're infected.

DID YOU KNOW?

Every year, about half of the people who get infected with hepatitis A never figure out where they got it.

ONE PERSON'S STORY

"Sometime in March, the food or water [Allison] ingested was contaminated with infected feces. It could have happened in Seattle or Bellingham, where she was checking out colleges. It could have happened after golf team practices at any burger joint that offers immediate relief to gnawing stomachs. It could have happened at a grocery store or even a friend's house. Allison will never know. By the time she was diagnosed three weeks ago, the virus had incubated in her for two months. Tracking its origins was impossible."

Source: Taggart, Cynthia. "Virus Saps Grad in Her Peak Weeks." *Spokesman-Review*, June 7, 1998. https://www.immunize.org/wp-content/uploads /reports/report013.pdf.

What Are the Symptoms of Hepatitis A?

The severity of illness is determined by age. Only about 30 of 100 children younger than six years old will have symptoms during infection; however, about 70 of 100 older children and adults will experience symptoms of the disease, which can include:

- Fever
- Feeling "out of sorts"
- Jaundice (yellowing of the skin and eyes)
- Dark-colored urine
- Abdominal pain
- Lack of appetite or aversion to food
- Nausea

Some people suffer severe, overwhelming infection with massive liver damage. About 15 of 100 people infected with hepatitis A virus require hospitalization. Before the vaccine, every year about seventy people in the United States died from hepatitis A infection.

DID YOU KNOW?

Although most young children don't develop symptoms during hepatitis A infection, they can still transmit the virus to others. Before the vaccine was routinely recommended for children, young children in day cares and those in contact with them were among the highest-risk groups. In 2006, the hepatitis A vaccine was recommended for routine use in children during their second year of life. Within five years of that recommendation, cases of hepatitis A dropped by about 95 percent.

HEPATITIS A: THE VACCINE
What Is the Hepatitis A Vaccine?

Two hepatitis A vaccines are available in the United States: Vaqta and Havrix. Both are made from hepatitis A virus grown in fetal embryo cells (see "Are Vaccines Made Using Aborted Fetal Cells?"). The vaccine virus is then completely inactivated with formaldehyde (see "Do Vaccines Contain Harmful Chemicals

Like Formaldehyde?"). Both vaccines also contain aluminum salts to enhance the immune response (see "Do Vaccines Contain Harmful Adjuvants Like Aluminum?").

Who Should Get the Hepatitis A Vaccine?

All children between twelve and twenty-three months of age are recommended to receive two doses of hepatitis A vaccine separated by six months. Children between two and eighteen years of age who haven't received the hepatitis A vaccine should also get vaccinated.

Several groups of adults are at increased risk of hepatitis A and are therefore recommended to get two or three doses, depending on the vaccine used. These groups include those with chronic liver disease, those with HIV, men who have sex with men, people who use drugs, people experiencing homelessness, people traveling internationally to countries with moderate or high rates of hepatitis A, close contacts of international adoptees, and those whose occupation increases their risk, such as those who work with some of the aforementioned groups. If you are unsure whether you would be considered high risk, talk with your health care provider. However, any adults who have not been vaccinated against hepatitis A but want to be protected can be vaccinated. Most hepatitis A vaccines are given in two doses, but if individuals eighteen years of age or older receive the combination hepatitis A and hepatitis B vaccine called Twinrix, they will need three doses.

Does the Hepatitis A Vaccine Work?

About 95 of 100 people who get the hepatitis A vaccine will be protected from infection.

Who Should Delay or Avoid Getting Hepatitis A Vaccine?

Those with moderate or severe illness should delay getting immunized until they are better, and anyone with a previous severe allergic reaction to a hepatitis A vaccine or any of its ingredients should not get additional doses.

What Are the Side Effects of Hepatitis A Vaccine?

People who have received hepatitis A vaccine may experience minor side effects:

- Pain, redness, or swelling at the injection site occurs in about 35 of 100 people.
- Mild fever or feeling tired or "out of sorts" occurs in fewer than five of 100 people.

Why Get the Hepatitis A Vaccine?

1. *It's hard to know who's contagious.* People tend to spread hepatitis A virus one to two weeks *before* they have symptoms. Also, many young children infected with the virus don't develop symptoms but are still contagious.
2. *Common activities like eating at a restaurant can lead to infection with hepatitis A.* One of the worst outbreaks of hepatitis A infection occurred at a Mexican restaurant in western Pennsylvania. About six hundred people were infected, and four died. The outbreak was eventually traced to green onions imported from Mexico that had not been washed properly.
3. *Hepatitis A infections can last a long time.* Most have symptoms that last about two months, but some suffer symptoms for as long as six months.
4. *People die from hepatitis A infections.* Between 2016 and May of 2023, more than four hundred people in the United States died from hepatitis A.
5. *The vaccine is safe.* Although some minor side effects occur, the vaccine is remarkably safe.

HEPATITIS A: OTHER THINGS YOU MIGHT HAVE WONDERED ABOUT

History of Hepatitis A Vaccine

The hepatitis A vaccine became available in 1995 and was first recommended for children living in states with the highest rates of hepatitis A, specifically, those with at least twice the national average. These states were primarily located in the west and southwest. The recommendation was expanded in 1999 to include children living in states, counties, or communities with rates of hepatitis A higher than the national average, even if less than twice as high. In 2006, the vaccine was recommended for all children between twelve and twenty-three months old because it was working well and because unimmunized communities were emerging as leaders in rates of hepatitis A disease. Since 1995, the incidence of hepatitis A infection in the United States has decreased dramatically. Unfortunately, outbreaks continue to occur, and, in some cases, the virus lingers in communities for many months, spreading from individual to individual, ultimately causing more cases than caused by the original outbreak.

Hepatitis A and International Travel

Many areas of the world still have large numbers of people infected with hepatitis A; in fact, it's one of the most common vaccine-preventable diseases acquired during travel.

While the risk of hepatitis A infection depends on travel conditions, such as length of stay, sanitary conditions (particularly in places where people eat), and activities (e.g., trekking in backwoods or rural areas), many travelers who get hepatitis A frequent standard tourist areas. Talk with your health care provider or a travel clinic if you or your family will be traveling internationally, especially if you have an infant who hasn't yet received hepatitis A vaccine.

THINGS TO DO

If you are preparing to travel, check with your health care provider or a travel clinic about the hepatitis A vaccine. You can learn more about how to avoid infection with hepatitis A while traveling by consulting the CDC's travel website: https://wwwnc.cdc.gov/travel.

THINGS TO DO

Because internationally adopted children may have hepatitis A, they can transmit the disease to others when they arrive in the United States. Therefore, immunization is recommended for those traveling to get the child as well as anyone who will have close contact with the child after they return.

Recent Hepatitis A Outbreaks

Before the vaccine became available in the United States in 2005, 27,000 people got hepatitis A every year; in 2008, only 2,300 people got the disease. Although most cases were not related, some recent outbreaks have occurred:

- In 2013, 165 people in ten states got hepatitis A from contaminated pomegranate seeds used in an antioxidant blend.
- In 2016, 143 people across nine states got hepatitis A virus from contaminated frozen strawberries, and fifty-six of them required hospitalization.
- In 2019, twenty people from seven states got hepatitis A from contaminated fresh blackberries, and eleven of them were hospitalized.
- In 2022, nineteen people across four states were infected by eating contaminated fresh strawberries, and thirteen of them were hospitalized.
- Since 2016, thousands of people have been affected by ongoing transmission of hepatitis A virus. Cases have been reported in thirty-seven states, and several hundred people have died. Many of these outbreaks have been associated with people experiencing homelessness and drug use. However, the virus can and has spread to other members of some of the surrounding communities.

Hepatitis A: Additional Resources

ONLINE INFORMATION

"Hepatitis A": https://www.vaccineinformation.org/diseases/hepatitis-a/

"Hepatitis A Vaccine": https://www.voicesforvaccines.org/vaccine
-information/hepatitisa/

"Hepatitis A: What You Should Know": https://media.chop.edu/data
/files/pdfs/vaccine-education-center-hepatitis-a.pdf

"A Look at Each Vaccine: Hepatitis A Vaccine": https://www.chop.edu
/centers-programs/vaccine-education-center/vaccine-details/hepatitis
-a-vaccine

PHOTOS

"Hepatitis A Photos": https://www.vaccineinformation.org/photos
/hepatitis-a/

PERSONAL EXPERIENCES

"Parents PACK Personal Stories – Hepatitis A": https://www.chop.edu
/centers-programs/parents-pack/personal-stories/hepatitis

"Unprotected People Stories: Hepatitis A": https://www.immunize.org
/clinical/vaccine-confidence/unprotected-people/topic/hepa/

VACCINES FOR THREE- TO SIX-YEAR-OLDS

Between the ages of three and six years, children receive additional doses of vaccines they've received previously. Many of these doses are recommended around four years of age when the child is preparing to start school. These additional vaccine doses boost the child's immune system so that they are well prepared for possible exposure to several potentially dangerous pathogens.

VACCINES TO REVISIT
DTaP Vaccine
Children are recommended to get a fifth dose of the diphtheria, tetanus, and pertussis (DTaP) vaccine between four and six years of age. See the "Diphtheria, Tetanus, and Pertussis" section of the "Vaccines in the First Year of Life" chapter for details about these diseases and the DTaP vaccine.

Influenza Vaccine
Usually by the third year of life, a child has had at least two doses of influenza vaccine; however, if they have not, they may need to get two doses in one season. After having two doses of influenza

vaccine, children in this age group, like those older than them, are recommended to get one dose annually. To get more details about influenza and the vaccine, check the "Influenza" section of the "Vaccines in the First Year of Life" chapter.

Polio Vaccine

Children are recommended to get their final dose of polio vaccine at four years of age. To find out more about polio and the vaccine, refer to the "Polio" section of the "Vaccines in the First Year of Life" chapter.

MMR Vaccine

A second dose of measles-mumps-rubella (MMR) vaccine is recommended at four years of age. See the "Measles, Mumps, and Rubella" section of the "Vaccines in the Second Year of Life" chapter for details about these diseases and the MMR vaccine.

Chickenpox Vaccine

A second dose of chickenpox vaccine is also recommended at four years of age. To find out more about chickenpox and the vaccine, see the "Chickenpox" section of the "Vaccines in the Second Year of Life" chapter.

VACCINES FOR SEVEN- TO EIGHTEEN- YEAR-OLDS

VACCINES TO REVISIT

During children's adolescent and teen years, they will revisit some vaccines they received as younger children, and they will have an opportunity to be protected against some additional diseases. Vaccines given during this period of life serve one of three goals.

First, some vaccines boost existing immunity, which may have faded over time. Adolescents and teen have typically had these vaccine before, such as tetanus, diphtheria, pertussis, and influenza.

Second, some vaccines protect against pathogens that adolescents and teens are less likely to have been exposed to when they were younger, like human papillomavirus (HPV), which is transmitted by sexual contact. Even if your child probably won't be intimate with someone for several years, they will likely do so eventually. Since the vaccine creates better immunity at younger ages, generates long-lasting immunity, and works only when given before exposure to HPV, it's best to get this one out of the way early in adolescence.

Third, some vaccines are given because the risk of infection increases in the teen years, such as meningococcus. Young infants and teens are at the greatest risk from these infections, but teens tend to be in settings and engage in social behaviors that increase the likelihood of infection, such as sharing utensils or drinks with peers, going to sleepaway camp, and starting college. Another vaccine given to some adolescents and teens, depending on where they live, is the dengue vaccine. In this case, they must have proof of previous infection to get the vaccine. Dengue is discussed in greater detail later in this chapter.

Influenza Vaccine

Influenza vaccine is recommended annually for adolescents and teens. To get more details about influenza and the vaccine, check the "Influenza" section of the "Vaccines in the First Year of Life" chapter.

Tdap Vaccine

Adolescents are recommended to get another dose of diphtheria, tetanus, and pertussis vaccine at eleven years of age. The vaccine recommended at this age is slightly different from the version given earlier in childhood (DTaP). The vaccine for adolescents (and adults) is referred to as "Tdap" because it contains lower quantities of diphtheria and pertussis antigens (the parts of a vaccine that generate immunity), hence the lowercase "d" and "p" in the name. See the "Diphtheria, Tetanus, and Pertussis" section of the "Vaccines in the First Year of Life" chapter for more details about the Tdap vaccine and the diseases it protects against.

MENINGOCOCCUS

MENINGOCOCCUS: THE DISEASE

Meningococcus is a bacterium that causes two serious infections: meningitis and sepsis. Perhaps no disease is more devastating than meningococcal sepsis. Parents who have lost children to this disease tell similar stories: their child was fine one minute and dead only a few hours later.

ONE PERSON'S STORY

"Ryan had just graduated high school, reached pro golf status and was preparing for college. Meningococcal meningitis took his life in less than fourteen hours after the first onset of complaints and signs of an earache and a fever."

Source: Milley, Frankie. "Ryan Wayne Milley (Bear)." Meningitis Angels. Accessed September 3, 2023, at http://www.meningitis-angels.org/ryan-wayne-milley.html. (Frankie Milley is the founder of Meningitis Angels, a parent advocacy group: www.meningitis-angels.org.)

What Is Meningococcus?

Meningococcus is a bacterium covered by a complex sugar, called a polysaccharide. Five types of meningococcus most commonly cause disease in people: A, B, C, Y, and W-135. In the United States, types B, C, and Y account for most cases. But type B accounts for at least half of all cases in children younger than one year of age.

DID YOU KNOW?

Type A meningococcus used to be the most common cause of disease in sub-Saharan Africa (but was very rare in the United
(continued on next page)

(continued from previous page)

> States). However, since the introduction of a group A meningo-
> coccus vaccine in that region in 2010, epidemics of this type of
> meningococcus have disappeared.

Meningococcal bacteria live harmlessly on the lining of the
nose and throat in about one of every 10 people, but rates can
be as high as one of every four people. Most people who first
encounter meningococcus never become sick, but they can still
transmit the deadly infection to others, primarily through respiratory secretions, for example, by sharing a glass or kissing.

Who Is Most Likely to Get a Meningococcal Infection?

Before the meningococcal vaccine first became available in the
United States in 2005, the group most likely to catch meningococcus was children less than two years of age; about seven of one
hundred thousand children under two years of age suffered meningococcus every year. The next group most likely to be infected was
adolescents and teens; about two of one hundred thousand of this
group caught it. Although the disease is more common in young
children, deaths are more common in teenagers.

Other groups at high risk for meningococcal disease include:

- People who have recently had a viral infection of the nose, throat,
  or lungs
- First-year college students living in dorms
- Military recruits living in barracks
- People exposed to tobacco smoke or indoor wood-burning stoves
- People who go to bars or nightclubs
- People who share drinking glasses or cigarettes
- People who binge drink

These groups are at highest risk because they have either
recently experienced a disruption of their throat lining (from

having a respiratory virus or by drinking or smoking), making it easier for meningococcal bacteria that occasionally live on the back of the throat to enter the bloodstream, or they are in close contact with others (in dorms or barracks), making it easier for the bacteria to travel from one person to another.

Some other groups are at increased risk because of their immune system status. These groups include people with complement deficiencies (complement proteins help the body fight infections) those without a spleen or with a spleen that does not work properly, and those with HIV/AIDS or sickle cell disease. Men who have sex with men tend to be at increased risk, possibly because of infections, like HIV, that affect the immune system, and people who work with bacteria in a laboratory are also at increased risk.

What Are the Symptoms of Meningococcus?

Meningococcus causes several types of infections:

- *Meningitis.* An infection of the lining of the brain and spinal cord, meningitis occurs in about half of people with meningococcal disease. Symptoms are similar to those of meningitis caused by other infections and include fever, headache, seizures, and stiff neck. People with meningitis may also experience nausea, vomiting, sensitivity to light, and confusion. About 30 of 100 people will die from the infection. Several other bacteria can also cause meningitis, including pneumococcus and *Haemophilus influenzae* type b (Hib), which are also vaccine preventable.
- *Bloodstream infection (sepsis).* Fewer than half of those with a meningococcal infection will develop a bloodstream infection. Symptoms include sudden fever, rash that resembles bleeding under the skin (spots may be as small as a pinpoint), drop in blood pressure, shock, and organ failure. About 40 of 100 people will die from the infection.
- *Pneumonia.* About five to 10 of 100 people will experience an infection of the lungs caused by meningococcal bacteria.

Of those who survive meningococcal meningitis or sepsis, about 20 of 100 will be permanently harmed, suffering the amputation of an arm or leg, hearing loss, brain damage, kidney failure, or severe scarring of the skin.

MENINGOCOCCUS: THE VACCINE
What Is the Meningococcal Vaccine?

Three meningococcal vaccines are available:

- *MenACWY.* This vaccine is made by stripping the sugar coating (called a polysaccharide) from four types of meningococcal bacteria (A, C, Y, and W-135) and linking each to a harmless protein. For this reason, the vaccine is known as a conjugate vaccine.
- *MenB.* This vaccine is made by inserting genes from two or four surface proteins on the meningococcal B bacterium into a harmless type of *E. coli* bacteria so that as *E. coli* reproduces, the meningococcal B proteins are also produced. The meningococcal B proteins are then purified for the vaccine. This method of making a vaccine is known as recombinant vaccine technology.
- *MenABCWY.* This vaccine was approved by the FDA in late 2023. It contains conjugated polysaccharides (sugar coating) from meningococcus A, C, W, and Y and two proteins from meningococcus B. The components are made using a combination of conjugate and recombinant vaccine technologies as described for the two other meningococcal vaccines. This vaccine can be used for routine vaccination of those between 16 and 23 years of age when both MenACWY and MenB vaccines are needed during the same visit and for those 10 years and older who are at high risk for meningococcus and are due to get both vaccines.

DID YOU KNOW?

The meningococcal B vaccine is made differently from the meningococcal ACWY vaccine for a couple of reasons. First, the type B polysaccharide did not produce a strong enough immune response even when attached to a helper protein (conjugate). Second, the type B polysaccharide has similarities to a human protein, so there was a chance that antibodies generated against a type B polysaccharide vaccine could cross-react with the human protein. Therefore, scientists had to pursue a different approach for making a meningococcal B vaccine.

Who Should Get the Meningococcal Vaccine?

Two doses of meningococcal ACWY (MenACWY) vaccine are recommended for adolescents and teens. The first should be given between eleven and twelve years of age, and the second should be given at sixteen years of age. This vaccine is also recommended for thirteen- to eighteen-year-olds who haven't had it yet. The number of doses depends on the age at which the vaccine is given.

People at higher risk of meningococcal disease should also be immunized, including those who:

- Do not have a spleen due to injury or do not have a working spleen due to sickle cell disease
- Have certain immune deficiencies
- Plan to travel to countries with high rates of meningococcal disease

In some situations, high-risk individuals require periodic booster doses of MenACWY vaccine.

Meningococcal B vaccine (MenB) can benefit anyone between sixteen and twenty-three years of age because they are all susceptible to this pathogen. However, it is recommended that caregivers and health care providers decide together whether an individual should get the vaccine and when. This "shared clinical decision-making" is recommended because protection lasts only for a year or two following vaccination, infection rates are typically low, and certain groups are at higher risk of infection than others (e.g., those living in college dorms or military barracks). For those who choose to get this vaccine, the preferred age is between sixteen and eighteen years. Two doses separated by one month or six months, depending on brand of vaccine, are recommended.

As with the types of meningococcus in the MenACWY vaccine, some individuals are at higher risk of meningococcal B infection, including those without a working spleen, those with certain immune-compromising conditions, and people traveling to certain locations.

DID YOU KNOW?

Meningococcal disease occurs so commonly in sub-Saharan Africa between Eritrea in the east and Senegal in the west that the area is referred to as the "meningitis belt." Epidemics of disease occur in this region between December and June. For this reason, the government of Saudi Arabia requires meningococcal ACWY immunization for travelers to Mecca for the Muslim pilgrimages of Hajj and Umrah.

Does the Meningococcal Vaccine Work?

About 70 of 100 people immunized with the MenACWY vaccine will develop protective immunity, and about 85 of 100 people immunized with the MenB vaccine will be protected.

Who Should Delay or Avoid Getting the Meningococcal Vaccine?

Those who have had a severe allergic reaction to a previous dose of meningococcal vaccine or one of its ingredients should not get additional doses of the same type of vaccine. Because of how the vaccines are made, people with a severe allergic reaction to a previous dose of a diphtheria-toxoid- or diphtheria-protein-based vaccine should not get the MenACWY vaccines known as Menveo or Menactra, and those with a severe allergic reaction to a previous dose of a tetanus-toxoid-based vaccine should not get MenQuadfi or Penbraya.

Anyone who is moderately or severely ill should delay getting immunized. Babies born prematurely who are at increased risk of meningococcal infection should not be given the MenACWY vaccine known as Menveo before nine months of age. Other brands may be used for individuals in this age group who require vaccination against meningococcus at a young age.

Pregnant people should delay getting the MenB vaccine if possible; however, the relative risks and benefits should be evaluated with one's health care provider.

What Are the Side Effects of the Meningococcal Vaccine?

Side effects of meningococcal vaccines include:

- Pain or redness at the injection site occurs in about 50 to 60 of 100 people.
- Fever of at least 100°F occurs in about five of 100 people.
- Headache, tiredness, or feeling "out of sorts" occurs in about 60 of 100 people.

Why Get Both Meningococcal Vaccines?

1. *People die from meningococcal disease every year in the United States.* Although rates of meningococcal disease have continued to decrease over time, every year some people get ill, and some die. The highest rates of disease are in young infants under the age of one year, but risk increases again during the late teens and early twenties and is also higher among aging adults.

2. *Meningococcal disease can't be predicted.* Only about five of 100 people with meningococcal disease were recently exposed to someone known to have been infected. The other 95 of 100 were exposed to someone who was carrying the bacteria in their nose and throat but was not infected by it.

3. *The vaccine will protect your child when you can't be there.* As adolescents and teens get older and become more social, they are at increased risk of infection. When they share water bottles on the football field, move into a college dorm, or go dancing at a bar

with friends, their risk increases. If they have had the vaccine, you can be assured that you have done what you can to protect them from this horrible disease.

4. *Many don't recover from meningococcal infections.* Even if your loved one survives a meningococcal infection, there is a good chance that their life may be changed forever because of permanent damage, such as amputations, hearing loss, or brain damage.

5. *The vaccine is safe.* While some side effects occur, they are relatively minor.

THINGS TO DO

Teenagers are more likely to faint after getting a vaccine than younger children; however, it can happen to anyone. If you or a family member is nervous about vaccination or faints easily, be sure to be seated or lying down for shots and wait at the doctor's office for about 15 minutes after being vaccinated.

MENINGOCOCCUS: OTHER THINGS YOU MIGHT HAVE WONDERED ABOUT

Meningococcal Vaccine and Guillain-Barré Syndrome

Guillain-Barré syndrome (GBS) is a disease characterized by weakened muscles, burning or tingling sensation in the legs or arms, loss of muscle tone, and sometimes paralysis. GBS occurs when a person's immune system attacks the proteins that line nerves. Although the exact cause is not known, some people get the disease after having a viral infection that affects the lungs or digestive tract. GBS is very rare, occurring in about one of one hundred thousand people every year.

Some adolescents have been diagnosed with GBS shortly after receiving meningococcal vaccine, so their parents have wondered whether the vaccine caused the disease. By the end of 2008, thirty-three people reported GBS following meningococcal vaccine to the Vaccine Adverse Event Reporting System (VAERS). In response, the CDC performed studies to determine whether GBS occurred more frequently in vaccinated people. It didn't. The incidence of GBS was the same in people who did and didn't receive the vaccine.

The meningococcal vaccine does not cause GBS.

> **THINGS TO DO**
>
> If a person has a history of GBS but also falls into a group at high risk for meningococcal disease, the vaccine is still recommended because the risk of GBS is theoretical (and arguably has been disproved), but the risk of meningococcal disease is real.

Infants, Types of Meningococcal Bacteria, and U.S. Vaccines

Despite the fact that children less than two years old are at the highest risk of getting meningococcal disease, current recommendations do not include routine use of meningococcal vaccines for those in this age group. This is because young children are most commonly infected with meningococcus type B, and, until relatively recently, no MenB vaccine was available. Although MenB vaccines are now available, young infants still are not routinely recommended to get these vaccines because of the low number of infections per year relative to the cost of vaccinating all children, waning immunity following vaccination, and limited data on the best approach for booster doses as children get older. Hopefully, at some point, this disease will also be routinely preventable in our youngest children.

Young Adults Who Don't Go to College or Who Go to College but Don't Live in Dorms

First-year college students living in dorms are at increased risk of getting infected with meningococcal bacteria, so they're recommended to have received the MenACWY vaccine within the last five years, preferably around sixteen years of age. Likewise, these individuals are at increased risk for meningococcal B infection, so they should also get the MenB vaccine between sixteen and eighteen years of age.

But, in reality, all young people are at increased risk compared with the general population beginning around fifteen years of age and extending through their early twenties. So, if your child did not receive the meningococcal vaccine as an adolescent and is not going to college or is not going to live in a college dorm or military barrack, you may still consider both of these vaccines. These vaccines are safe, and they can save lives.

Exposure to Meningococcus

When a case of meningococcal meningitis is reported in a community, people panic. Was my child exposed? Do I need to get antibiotics? It is both scary and confusing, so here's the scoop.

Although this disease is contagious, it is not the most contagious disease out there. Only about five of 100 cases occur during outbreaks; the rest occur singly and sporadically. That said, when someone has meningococcal meningitis or sepsis, certain people are at particularly high risk of getting infected from them, including:

- People who live with the infected person (a 500- to 800-fold higher risk)
- People who shared a classroom or workspace with the infected person during the week before the illness
- People who were directly exposed to the sick person's saliva through kissing, sharing utensils or toothbrushes, or administering medical care during the week before the illness
- People seated next to the infected person during a flight longer than eight hours

These people should receive antibiotics and possibly vaccination. People who did not have direct contact with the infected person do not require treatment. Local public health officials typically work to identify and contact those who require treatment.

Meningococcus: Additional Resources

ONLINE INFORMATION

"Can You Tell Me More About the Outbreaks of Meningitis on College Campuses?": https://www.chop.edu/centers-programs/vaccine-education-center/video/can-you-tell-me-more-about-outbreaks-meningitis-college-campuses

"Doctors Talk: Meningitis": https://www.chop.edu/centers-programs/vaccine-education-center/video/doctors-talk-meningitis

"A Look at Each Vaccine: Meningococcal Vaccine": https://www.chop.edu/centers-programs/vaccine-education-center/vaccine-details/meningococcal-vaccine

"Meningococcal Disease": https://www.vaccineinformation.org/diseases/meningococcal/

"Meningococcal Vaccines": https://www.voicesforvaccines.org/vaccine-information/meningitis/

"Meningococcus Vaccine–Why Do College Students Need It?":https://www.youtube.com/watch?v=7zinvvw9M8E

"Meningococcus: What You Should Know": https://media.chop.edu/data/files/pdfs/vaccine-education-center-meningococcus.pdf

Talking About Vaccines with Dr. Paul Offit: News Briefs – September 2016 – Meningococcus B Vaccine": https://www.chop.edu/video/talking-about-vaccines-dr-paul-offit-news-briefs-september-2016-meningococcus-b-vaccine

PHOTOS

"Meningococcal Photos": https://www.vaccineinformation.org/photos/meningococcal/

PERSONAL EXPERIENCES

"Parents PACK Personal Stories – Meningococcus": http://www.chop.edu/service/parents-possessing-accessing-communicating

-knowledge-about-vaccines/sharing-personal-stories/meningococcus
.html

"Story Gallery": https://www.shotbyshot.org/story-gallery/ (search "meningitis" and "meningitis type B")

"Unprotected People Stories: Meningococcal": https://www.immunize
.org/clinical/vaccine-confidence/unprotected-people/topic
/meningococcal/

SUPPORT GROUPS

Meningitis Angels: http://www.meningitis-angels.org/

American Society for Meningitis Prevention https://meningitis
prevention.org/

HUMAN PAPILLOMAVIRUS

HUMAN PAPILLOMAVIRUS: THE DISEASE

Human papillomavirus (HPV) infects cells that line the surfaces of our mouth, throat, and genital areas. If our immune system cannot overcome the infection, the virus persists, replicating for years in some people. Often, these individuals don't know they're infected. Over time, infected cells can transform, resulting in cancer. HPV infections are known to cause cancer in the throat, tongue, voice box, anus, penis, vulva, and vagina, as well as virtually all cases of cancer in the cervix, one of the most common cancers in women. In 2018, Dr. Tedros Adhanom Ghebreyesus, the director-general of the World Health Organization, stated, "One woman dies of cervical cancer every two minutes. . . . Each one is a tragedy, and we can prevent it." He was talking about the HPV vaccine.

ONE PERSON'S STORY

"My dad's life changed a lot. He had so many surgeries. There was one to take out a mass the doctors found in his neck, which turned out to be cancer. Then they took out his tonsils because they were looking for where the cancer was coming from. Then he had another one to insert a feeding tube in his stomach. He had four different operations to widen his throat. He also needed both "chemo" (chemotherapy) and radiation treatments to fight his cancer.

"Because of his cancer and treatments, my dad lost around thirty pounds. And he always looked pale white like he was really sick. The treatments to his throat made it so he couldn't swallow so he couldn't eat the normal way anymore. And the treatments made him lose his voice too. He also had to have a sucking tube down his throat that was always sucking up gunky mucus. He

(*continued on next page*)

(continued from previous page)

needed that because he couldn't swallow, and he would choke. It was a lot of stuff."

Source: "Matthew's Story." ShotByShot.org. Accessed September 19, 2023, at https://www.shotbyshot.org/stories/matthews-story/. Reprinted and excerpted with permission from ShotByShot.org.

What Is HPV?

HPV is a common infection of both men and women, spread from one person to another through sexual contact. About forty-two million Americans are currently infected with HPV, and thirteen million new infections occur every year. About 80 of 100 sexually active adults will have at least one HPV infection, and about 40 of 100 girls and women are infected within the first two years of becoming sexually active. Women can also transmit the virus to their newborn infants during childbirth, occasionally leading to a rare condition called recurrent respiratory papillomatosis (RRP).

ONE PERSON'S STORY

"Today, Emma is 7 years old and she has had two surgeries. Unfortunately, both surgeries have involved the most sensitive area of her vocal cords . . . and have left her with very limited and altered vocal ability. I have not heard my daughter laugh since before her second surgery 3½ months ago. She is physically unable. If you were not looking at her face, you would not know she is laughing. It absolutely breaks my heart. My daughter used to love to sing. Now, she is physically unable to sing. Not only because she barely has any vocal range, but because she is embarrassed at how awful her voice sounds. She used to love to read out loud to me, but now it is just a struggle for her. This is just the tip of the iceberg when it comes to ways my daughter's quality of life has been affected."

Source: Sinn, Kate. "My Beautiful Daughter Emma Was Diagnosed with RRP at the Age of 5½." Recurrent Respiratory Papillomatosis Foundation (www.RRPF.org or info@rrpf.org). Accessed September 30, 2023, at https://rrpf.org/emma-sinn/.

Unlike measles, mumps, rubella, and chickenpox, in which only one type of virus causes disease, more than one hundred types of HPV have been identified. Some HPV types are known as "high-risk" types because they can cause cancers of the cervix, head, neck, anus, vagina, vulva, and penis. Most people with HPV eliminate the infection without consequence and never know they were infected. However, some people remain infected for a long time, increasing their risk of getting cancer, which usually develops twenty to twenty-five years after the initial infection.

So-called "low-risk" types of HPV cause anal and genital warts, which can be disfiguring, painful, and emotionally upsetting. Every year, before an HPV vaccine was available, three hundred thousand to four hundred thousand Americans sought medical care for genital warts caused by HPV. This number is likely to be underestimated since not everyone with an infection seeks medical care. It's estimated that at any point in time, about one of every 100 sexually active adults in the United States have genital warts.

HUMAN PAPILLOMAVIRUS: THE VACCINE
What Is HPV Vaccine?

The HPV vaccine is made using recombinant technology, which involves taking the HPV gene that makes one protein from the surface of the virus and putting it inside a plasmid (a small circular piece of DNA that can reproduce inside cells). The plasmid is then put inside common baker's yeast, where it produces the viral surface protein. The protein is purified away from the yeast to make the vaccine. Interestingly, the protein assembles itself to look just like the virus, making it unique because although on the outside, it looks like natural HPV, there's one important difference: the inside is empty, meaning the vaccine doesn't contain viral DNA, so it can't possibly reproduce. These structures are called virus-like particles or VLPs. To enhance the immune response, the vaccine also contains aluminum salts that serve as an adjuvant (see "Do Vaccines Contain Harmful Adjuvants Like Aluminum?").

The current HPV vaccine used in the United States contains the HPV surface protein from the nine types of HPV that cause the most disease in people. Seven are high-risk, or cancer-causing, types, and two are low-risk types that cause genital warts but not cancer. The high-risk types contained in the vaccine include HPV types 16, 18, 31, 33, 45, 52, and 58. Types 16 and 18 are responsible for the largest number of HPV-related cancers in both men and women around the world, accounting for 70 to 80 of every 100 cases. The low-risk types included in the HPV-9 vaccine are types 6 and 11. Together, these two types cause 90 of every 100 cases of genital warts.

DID YOU KNOW?

The first HPV vaccine was approved in 2006, but it wasn't the first vaccine to prevent cancer in people. The first cancer-prevention vaccine was the hepatitis B vaccine, which prevents liver cancer.

Who Should Get HPV Vaccine?

The HPV vaccine is recommended for all adolescents between eleven and twelve years of age, but it can be given as early as nine years of age. Those up to twenty-six years of age who have not received the vaccine are also recommended to get it, and individuals between the ages of twenty-seven and forty-five years of age can discuss the potential risks and benefits of vaccination with their health care provider.

Most who get the HPV vaccine before they turn fifteen years old should get two doses separated by six to twelve months. Anyone fifteen years of age or older and those younger than fifteen years of age with certain immune-compromising conditions require three doses. The second dose should be given one to two months after the first dose, and the third dose should be given at least six months after the first dose.

Who Should Delay or Avoid Getting HPV Vaccine?

Anyone who has had a severe allergic reaction to a dose of HPV vaccine or any of its ingredients, including yeast, should not get future doses. Those who have moderate or severe illness should wait until they have recovered before getting vaccinated.

Does the HPV Vaccine Work?

The HPV vaccine prevents almost all long-lasting HPV infections that can lead to cancer. As a result, in the first decade after HPV vaccine became available, studies showed that infections with the types of HPV included in the vaccine decreased among those first recommended to get it. Teenage girls fourteen to nineteen years of age were almost 90 percent less likely to be infected, and women in their early twenties were almost 70 percent less likely to be infected.

Importantly, the HPV vaccine does not protect people against types of HPV to which they have previously been exposed. As such, getting adolescents vaccinated early is important for them to have the best opportunity for protection.

What Are the Side Effects of HPV Vaccine?

HPV vaccine is safe but can cause a few minor side effects:

- Pain, redness, or swelling at the injection site occurs in 20 to 90 of 100 people.

- Fainting occurs in about eight of one hundred thousand people.
- Allergic reactions occur in about one of one million people.

Why Get the HPV Vaccine?

1. *HPV is the most common sexually transmitted disease in the United States, causing thirteen million new infections every year.*

2. *The single best chance to protect against cancer caused by HPV is to get the vaccine before becoming sexually active.* That's because the vaccine only works to *prevent* the disease; it doesn't treat it. Because we don't know when our children will become sexually active, and because they get busier as they get older, it is better to get the vaccine earlier rather than later.

3. *People who are already sexually active can also benefit.* Even though a person might be infected by one or even a few types of HPV, it's unlikely that they would have already been infected with all nine types of HPV contained in the vaccine.

4. *The vaccine also protects against anal and genital warts.* While most people talk about the cancer prevention associated with HPV vaccination, it's worth remembering that the vaccine also protects against anal and genital warts. While not life-threatening, these growths can be disfiguring and cause a range of emotional consequences, including depression, anxiety, and decreased self-confidence.

5. *Greater use of the vaccine means less virus spread in the community.* If more people are immune to HPV, fewer will become infected and transmit the virus to their sexual partners. Protecting yourself or your child also protects future sexual partners.

6. *The vaccine is safe.* Although HPV vaccine has some mild side effects, none is severe or permanent.

HUMAN PAPILLOMAVIRUS: OTHER THINGS YOU MIGHT HAVE WONDERED ABOUT
HPV Vaccine Safety

Stories in the media, primarily personal accounts, have suggested that the HPV vaccine can cause debilitating illness and death. As mentioned, when a vaccine side effect is experienced, it can be reported to VAERS (see "What Systems Are in Place to Ensure That Vaccines Are Safe?"). These reports are investigated by public health officials who interview the individual or family and health care providers. They also review the affected person's medical chart. The investigators are interested in three things: why the individual experienced the reported event, whether it could have been caused by the vaccine, and whether other people vaccinated with the same vaccine have also had similar experiences. If the vaccine might be causing the problem, investigators will study large numbers of people who did and did not get the vaccine to see whether the vaccine and the side effect are related.

For example, although some young women have experienced blood clots, strokes, or heart attacks following receipt of the HPV vaccine, studies have shown that these problems were not caused by the vaccine. Rather, they were caused by a medication known to cause blood clots, strokes, and heart attacks: birth control pills. So, it's important to realize that while the stories of individuals are powerful, their experiences are not necessarily related to receipt of the vaccine, even if the two things occurred close in time.

Similarly, investigators have found that teenagers who have received HPV vaccine are not at greater risk of autoimmune or other conditions than those who haven't gotten the vaccine. Studies have evaluated numerous conditions, including GBS, chronic fatigue syndrome (CFS), multiple sclerosis (MS), chronic regional pain syndromes (CRPS), postural orthostatic tachycardia syndrome (POTS), and primary ovarian failure. (For summaries of some of these studies, visit the "HPV Vaccine Safety Concerns" section of the Vaccine Education Center at Children's Hospital of Philadelphia's "Vaccine Safety References" web page: https://www.chop.edu/centers-programs/vaccine-education-center/vaccine-safety-references.)

HPV and Pap Tests

Pap tests monitor for cellular changes in the cervix that suggest a long-term HPV infection. Once cells are isolated during an appointment, the sample is fixed to a microscope slide and viewed by someone experienced at identifying changes in cells of the cervix. These changes are referred to as cervical intraepithelial neoplasia (CIN), and they are graded according to how extensive they are. Three stages have been identified: CIN 1, 2, and 3. All people who eventually get cervical cancer pass through these three stages.

Some people wonder if they can forgo Pap tests if they've had the HPV vaccine. The short answer is no for a couple of reasons. First, people may have been infected before getting the vaccine. Since the vaccine does not work against prior infections, regular Pap tests can detect cellular changes that could occur because of any pre-vaccine infections. Second, while the HPV vaccine protects against most types of HPV that cause cancer, it does not protect against all of them, so Pap tests can still detect these rare cases of cancer. Third, while the vaccine protects virtually everyone who is vaccinated, it is possible that someone was not protected against one or more types of HPV in the vaccine. Pap tests can help in this scenario as well.

Males and HPV Vaccine

When the HPV vaccine was first introduced, it was recommended for females but not males. This gender-specific recommendation was made for a few reasons, including that the studies conducted until that point had been done primarily in females. However, shortly thereafter, studies in males showed the vaccine to be safe and effective in preventing anal and genital warts. In 2009, the vaccine became available for males, and since then, data have continued to show the benefits of HPV vaccination for males, including a decrease in cancers caused by HPV among males. About one-third of all HPV-related cancers occur in men. Current HPV vaccine recommendations do not differ between females and males, including the opportunity to be vaccinated up to forty-five years of age.

> **DID YOU KNOW?**
>
> One concern about the HPV vaccine was that it would increase sexual promiscuity. Studies have shown that not to be the case. Further, related evidence suggests that this would never have been an issue, even before the studies were completed:
>
> - Distribution of condoms and increased availability of the morning-after pill have not led to increases in sexual activity among adolescents and teens.
> - Avoiding sexually transmitted diseases is not why most teenagers choose to wait to have sex. Rather, the most common reasons are religious beliefs, wanting to avoid pregnancy, and absence of an appropriate partner.
> - Parental monitoring, one's peer group, the age of one's romantic partner, and television programming are the most influential factors in determining the age at which sexual activity begins.

Human Papillomavirus: Additional Resources

ONLINE INFORMATION

"Doctors Talk: HPV": https://www.chop.edu/centers-programs/vaccine-education-center/video/doctors-talk-hpv

"Human Papillomavirus": https://media.chop.edu/data/files/pdfs/human-papillomavirus-infographic.pdf

"Human Papillomavirus (HPV)": https://www.vaccineinformation.org/diseases/hpv/

"Human Papillomavirus (HPV) Vaccine": https://www.voicesforvaccines.org/vaccine-information/hpv/

"Human Papillomavirus: What You Should Know": https://media.chop.edu/data/files/pdfs/vaccine-education-center-hpv.pdf

"Is the HPV Vaccine Safe?": https://www.chop.edu/centers-programs
/vaccine-education-center/video/hpv-vaccine-safe

"A Look at Each Vaccine: Human Papillomavirus": https://www.chop
.edu/centers-programs/vaccine-education-center/vaccine-details
/human-papillomavirus

"Questions and Answers About HPV and the Vaccine": http://prevent
-HPV.org

"The Stages of Viral Infection: How HPV and Shingles Play a Long
Game": https://www.chop.edu/video/stages-viral-infection-how
-hpv-and-shingles-play-long-game

"Talking About Vaccines with Dr. Paul Offit: HPV (Human Papillomavirus)":   https://www.chop.edu/centers-programs/vaccine
-education-center/resources/vaccine-videos-and-dvds/hpv-human
-papillomavirus

"Talking About Vaccines with Dr. Paul Offit: News Briefs – August
2017 – HPV Vaccine and Chronic Diseases": https://www.chop.edu
/video/talking-about-vaccines-dr-paul-offit-news-briefs-august
-2017-hpv-vaccine-and-chronic-diseases

PHOTOS

"HPV Photos": https://www.cdc.gov/hpv/hcp/photos.html

PERSONAL EXPERIENCES

"Lady Ganga: Nilza's Story": https://www.youtube.com/watch?v
=u5yMCzxoctU

Someone You Love: The HPV Epidemic (documentary): https://hpvepidemic
.vhx.tv/

"Story Gallery": https://www.shotbyshot.org/story-gallery/ (search
"HPV all")

"Unprotected People Stories: HPV (Human Papillomavirus)": https://
www.immunize.org/clinical/vaccine-confidence/unprotected
-people/topic/hpv/

SUPPORT GROUPS

Cervivor: https://cervivor.org/

DENGUE

DENGUE: THE DISEASE

Dengue is a virus that is spread to people through the bite of a mosquito. About half the world's population, about four billion people, live in areas where dengue is common, specifically, the Americas, Africa, the Middle East, Asia, and the Pacific Islands. Dengue is common in the U.S. territories of American Samoa, Puerto Rico, and the U.S. Virgin Islands.

Every year, as many as four hundred million people get infected with dengue virus; about one hundred million get sick, and forty thousand die. Because there are four types of dengue virus (types 1, 2, 3, and 4), people can be infected as many as four times during their lifetime.

What Is Dengue?

Dengue is a virus. Four types of dengue virus can cause disease ranging from an asymptomatic or mild infection to a severe and occasionally fatal disease. People are much more likely to develop severe dengue the second time they are infected.

DID YOU KNOW?

Dengue also occurs in the continental United States. Recent outbreaks of dengue have occurred in Florida and Texas, as well as Hawaii.

THINGS TO DO

The mosquitoes that spread dengue virus to people are the same types that spread Zika and chikungunya viruses. These mosquitoes typically lay eggs near standing water or in containers that

(*continued on next page*)

(continued from previous page)

hold water. They bite people both during the day and at night. Mosquitoes become infected with dengue virus when they bite people who are infected with it. They then transmit the virus when they bite other people.

People can best avoid mosquito bites by using insect repellents approved by the Environmental Protection Agency (EPA), such as those containing DEET, Picaridin, IR3535, oil of lemon eucalyptus, para-menthane-diol, or 2-undecanone.

What Are the Symptoms of Dengue?

Dengue is defined by a combination of two or more clinical symptoms in a person with fever who has recently traveled to an area where dengue is common. Symptoms include nausea, vomiting, rash, aches and pains, a low white blood cell count, and evidence of easy bleeding, such as unexplained bleeding from the nose or gums, vomiting blood, or having blood in one's feces. Severe dengue is defined by symptoms including shock, severe bleeding, liver disease, impaired consciousness, or heart disease.

About one in four people infected with dengue virus will experience symptoms. The early phase of dengue infection is characterized by fever lasting two to seven days; severe headache; eye pain; muscle, joint, and bone pain; rash; and evidence of bleeding from the skin and gums. Some people then progress to more severe disease, characterized by shock and massive bleeding. About one of 20 people with dengue will develop severe disease.

DID YOU KNOW?

A pregnant person with dengue virus can transmit the virus to the unborn child, causing early delivery or fetal death. The pregnant person is also at increased risk for complications, including fever, increased fluid in the abdomen or between the lungs and chest wall, and bleeding disorders.

ONE PERSON'S STORY

"'I know that the more times you get dengue, the more serious it can get. So, of course I'm scared. The first time I just had a fever, but the second time my blood result was worrying. So, I'm scared of what will happen if I get it a third time.' Jhii also particularly worries about her daughter. 'She's so young. For me having been infected twice, there's a very high risk of her getting it. I just can't imagine a baby contracting dengue.'"

Source: Lian, Tan Jhii. "Living with Dengue: It's Everywhere and There's Nothing We Can Do About It." DNDi (Drugs for Neglected Diseases Initiative). January 26, 2022. https://dndi.org/stories/2022/living-with-dengue-its-everywhere-and-theres-nothing-we-can-do-about-it/.

DENGUE: THE VACCINE

What Is the Dengue Vaccine?

The dengue vaccine is a modified form of the yellow fever vaccine. To make the dengue vaccine, researchers took the yellow fever vaccine, which has been available for decades, and substituted genes that serve as a blueprint for two dengue virus proteins, the fusion protein and the envelope protein, into that vaccine. These two dengue virus proteins evoke antibodies that neutralize the virus. The dengue vaccine includes four combination viruses that protect against the four types of dengue.

The problem with dengue virus is that people are much more likely to suffer severe infection after their second exposure to the virus. Unfortunately, the same thing happened upon exposure to the virus after vaccination. Specifically, researchers found that when people who had never been infected before were vaccinated and later exposed to the virus, they, too, had more severe infection; the same thing that happens when people are exposed to the virus twice. During the vaccine study, vaccinated people who had never been exposed to the virus fared more poorly than unvaccinated people who had not been infected before. However, people who had been infected before vaccination had no problem with vaccination, nor did they suffer more severe disease when they had a subsequent encounter with the natural virus. For this reason, the dengue vaccine is recommended only for people who have previously been infected.

Who Should Get the Dengue Vaccine?

The dengue vaccine, Dengvaxia, is only recommended for certain people in the United States based on their age and where they live. Specifically, vaccination is recommended for those between nine and sixteen years of age who meet two criteria:

- They have been previously infected with dengue virus, as determined by clinical testing.
- They live in a high-risk area, such as the U.S. territories and freely associated states of American Samoa, Puerto Rico, U.S. Virgin Islands, Federated States of Micronesia, Republic of the Marshall Islands, or the Republic of Palau.

The dengue vaccine is given as a series of three doses. The second dose is given six months after the first dose, and the third dose is given twelve months after the first dose.

Who Should Avoid or Delay Getting the Dengue Vaccine?

Anyone less than nine years of age, anyone older than sixteen years of age, and anyone nine to sixteen years of age who has not previously been infected with dengue virus should not get the dengue vaccine. Those who have had a severe allergic reaction to a previous dose of the vaccine or to one of its ingredients and those with certain severe immune-compromising conditions should also avoid this vaccine.

Those who are pregnant, those with HIV who are not severely immune suppressed, and those with moderate or severe illness should discuss the relative risks and benefits of vaccination with their health care provider.

The dengue vaccine is not approved for U.S. travelers who are visiting but not living in areas where dengue is common.

Does the Dengue Vaccine Work?

The dengue vaccine protects 80 to 85 of 100 people from symptomatic infection, including severe disease. Protection lasts for at least six years.

What Are the Side Effects of the Dengue Vaccine?

The most frequently reported side effects of the dengue vaccine are headache, pain at the injection site, malaise, and muscle aches.

Why Get the Dengue Vaccine?

1. *Dengue is a severe and often fatal infection.* For those who live in areas where the virus is common, the dengue vaccine provides a high level of protection against serious disease with minimal side effects.
2. *A second infection with dengue is likely to be more severe than the first.* Given that we cannot always prevent mosquito bites and that second infections are worse, it's better to get vaccinated than experience the disease.
3. *The vaccine is safe and effective in those for whom it is recommended.*

DENGUE: OTHER THINGS YOU MIGHT HAVE WONDERED ABOUT
Dengue and COVID-19

Because the early symptoms of dengue and COVID-19 can be similar, it might be difficult to tell which infection someone has if they live in an area where dengue is common or if they recently traveled to such an area. In both infections, most cases are mild, and people can usually recover at home without medical intervention. However, if a person develops a severe case of either, it can be fatal, so health care providers need to monitor symptoms carefully and order tests to determine the cause of infection if warranted.

Severe dengue tends to occur more often, but not always, in infants and young children, whereas severe COVID-19 tends to occur more often, but not always, in older adults. Those with diabetes and chronic heart conditions are at increased risk from both infections.

Dengue: Additional Resources

ONLINE INFORMATION

"Dengue": https://www.cdc.gov/dengue/index.html

"Dengue": https://www.vaccineinformation.org/diseases/dengue/

"Dengue and Severe Dengue": https://www.who.int/news-room/fact-sheets/detail/dengue-and-severe-dengue

"A Look at Each Vaccine: Dengue Vaccine": https://www.chop.edu/centers-programs/vaccine-education-center/vaccine-details/look-each-vaccine-dengue

PHOTOS

CDC Public Health Image Library: https://phil.cdc.gov/Default.aspx (search "dengue")

VACCINES FOR ADULTS

VACCINES TO REVISIT

Some adults may realize they need certain vaccines, like the "flu" vaccine, "pneumonia vaccine," or shingles vaccine, but often, even if they know about vaccines, they don't take the time to get them. And in many cases, subgroups of adults don't even realize there are vaccines recommended for them. For example, are you aware of the following?

- Pregnant people should get a Tdap vaccine during a certain period of every pregnancy.
- People who smoke are recommended to get a pneumococcal vaccine.
- Every adult between nineteen and fifty-nine years of age is recommended to get a hepatitis B vaccine if they have not already had one. And those aged sixty years and older can get this vaccine if they want to protect themselves against hepatitis B.
- People sixty years of age and older are recommended to receive a vaccine to prevent respiratory syncytial virus (RSV), which, like influenza virus, can cause severe pneumonia.

Over time, the opportunities for adults to protect themselves against infectious diseases have increased.

Influenza Vaccine

Influenza vaccine is recommended annually for most adults, even those with egg allergies and those who have had Guillain-Barré syndrome (GBS). If GBS occurred in the six-week period following receipt of influenza vaccine, the individual has what is known as a "precaution" for future doses. In this scenario, it's worth talking with your health care provider about the relative risks and benefits of getting influenza vaccine. Unfortunately, many people—and even some health care providers—think that having a history of GBS means you can't get influenza vaccine, which is not accurate. To get more details about influenza and the vaccine, check the "Influenza" section of the "Vaccines in the First Year of Life" chapter.

Tdap or Td Vaccine

Adults are recommended to get the Tdap or Td vaccine every ten years throughout life to boost their immunity to tetanus and diphtheria. They can also boost their immunity to pertussis by asking for Tdap instead of Td. In a few situations, adults are recommended to get this vaccine even if it has been less than ten years since their last dose:

- *Never vaccinated against one or more of these pathogens or never had one dose of Tdap*: The number of doses a person needs depends on their situation. Talk with your health care provider if you are in either of these situations.
- *During every pregnancy*: The Tdap vaccine (not Td) is recommended between twenty-seven and thirty-six weeks of gestation during every pregnancy. By getting vaccinated, antibodies against pertussis (whooping cough) will cross the placenta and be transferred to the baby so that at birth and in the months thereafter, the baby will have some protection against this disease, which can be

fatal in the youngest among us. By the time the maternal antibodies wane, the baby will be getting their own vaccines and generating their own immunity.

- *During wound care*: When a person has a wound that requires medical care, they're often asked when their most recent tetanus vaccination was. In most cases, the person will be offered Tdap or Td if their last dose was more than five years ago or if they're not certain. If you're in this situation, you may want to check which type the health care provider plans to give and ask for Tdap instead of Td to boost your protection against pertussis.

See the "Diphtheria, Tetanus, and Pertussis" section of the "Vaccines in the First Year of Life" chapter for more details about the Tdap and Td vaccines and the diseases they protect against.

COVID-19 Vaccine

While most adults have been vaccinated against COVID-19, many have not. And, although the public health emergency was declared over in May 2023, the virus that causes COVID-19 will likely remain for decades to come. In the last months of the pandemic, most people being hospitalized and dying from COVID-19 were those who remained unvaccinated. As such, adults who have not been vaccinated against COVID-19 should reconsider.

Immunologic memory following receipt of COVID-19 vaccine has held up remarkably well, meaning that most people who have had some combination of doses of the vaccine will be protected against severe disease that results in hospitalization or death. However, studies have shown that a few subgroups could benefit from an additional booster dose, including those over sixty-five years of age, those with a compromised immune system, those with health conditions that increase their risk of severe infection, and pregnant people.

It's likely that COVID-19 vaccines and the recommendations for their use will evolve in the next few years as we learn more about SARS-CoV-2, the virus that causes COVID-19.

Hepatitis B Vaccine

Adults up to fifty-nine years of age who have not previously been vaccinated against hepatitis B are recommended to do so. Those sixty years of age and older in high-risk categories are also recommended to get this vaccine if they have not previously had it. Adults sixty years of age and older who are not considered to be high risk may also consider getting vaccinated to protect themselves against this virus. To find out who is at increased risk, learn more about hepatitis B virus, and get information about the vaccine, see the "Hepatitis B" section in the "Vaccines in the First Year of Life" chapter.

Pneumococcal Vaccine

As people age, their risk of infection with pneumococcal bacteria increases. This is due to changes in the immune system as people age. Pneumococcus is a particularly "opportunistic" pathogen in that it waits to strike until a person is run down from something else, particularly a respiratory viral infection like influenza. This is why you hear stories of adults starting to recover from a viral illness and then suddenly getting worse again, often becoming severely ill and ending up with pneumonia, being hospitalized, or even dying. Pneumococcus is very often to blame in these situations. It is for this reason that adults are recommended to get vaccinated against pneumococcus when they reach sixty-five years of age or as soon as possible if they are older than that. Some younger adults are also recommended to get this vaccine, such as those who smoke and those with certain chronic medical conditions, including alcoholism. For more information about pneumococcus and the vaccines to prevent it, see the "Pneumococcus" section of the "Vaccines in the First Year of Life" chapter.

Human Papillomavirus Vaccine

Adults can get the human papillomavirus (HPV) vaccine until forty-five years of age. Those younger than twenty-six years of age are recommended to do so, and those between twenty-six and forty-five years of age who have not yet been vaccinated should talk to their health care provider about the relative benefits of getting the vaccine. While the vaccine is less effective among older adults, it can still be of benefit because most people have not been exposed to all nine types of HPV contained in the vaccine. The decreased effectiveness is thought to be the result of previous HPV infections in older people since the vaccine does not protect against infections that occurred before vaccination, and people are more likely to have been infected with one or more types after they become sexually active. For more information about HPV and the vaccine, see the "Human Papillomavirus" section of the "Vaccines for 7- to 18-year-olds" chapter.

Hepatitis A Vaccine

People often think of hepatitis A vaccine as a "travel vaccine," meaning it is needed only for those traveling to places where exposure to this virus is more likely. However, outbreaks of hepatitis A occur regularly in the United States, and they often start when someone infected with hepatitis A (often unknowingly) handles food that does not get cooked, later causing disease in an unsuspecting consumer. This can happen eating out at restaurants or from frozen or fresh foods from the grocery store.

Additionally, several groups of individuals are at increased risk for this infection, which in the last few years has been causing outbreaks resulting from person-to-person transmission in some settings, such as among people using injection drugs or experiencing homelessness. Other groups of adults, such as those in close contact with international adoptees and those working with other high-risk groups are also at greater risk of contracting hepatitis A. To find out more about this disease and the vaccines to prevent it, see the "Hepatitis A" section of the "Vaccines in the Second Year of Life" chapter.

Polio Vaccine

Adults born and raised in the United States are typically considered to be immune to poliovirus. However, some adults may not know their immune status and be at high risk because of travel, an outbreak, their occupation, or other circumstances. In these situations, they may need doses of polio vaccine. Even in situations where someone knows they were previously vaccinated, if they are at high-risk, they may get a single lifetime booster dose of the inactivated polio vaccine (IPV). For more information about these recommendations, the disease, and the vaccine, see the "Polio" section of the "Vaccines in the First Year of Life" chapter.

Meningococcal Vaccine

Some adults are at increased risk of meningococcal infection because of certain health conditions or activities, such as international travel to a location where this disease is more common. One example is those planning to travel to Africa for the annual Muslim pilgrimage known as the Hajj. If you're not sure of your risk, talk with your health care provider. For more information about this disease and the vaccines that prevent it, see the "Meningococcus" section of the "Vaccines for 7- to 18-year-olds" chapter.

SHINGLES

SHINGLES: THE DISEASE

Shingles is a painful skin eruption that occurs in older adults and in people taking immune-suppressive medicines. The disease is five to ten times more likely to occur in people over sixty years of age and is more common in women than men. The disease is less common in Black people.

What Is Shingles?

After a natural infection with chickenpox (varicella), the virus lives silently in the nerve roots near the spine. In other words, you never completely rid yourself of the chickenpox virus after a natural infection.

Shingles is a disease caused by the reactivation of chickenpox virus from the central nervous system. Anyone who has been infected with chickenpox is at risk of shingles. For children infected with chickenpox in the first two years of life, the incidence of shingles is greater than for those infected at an older age.

DID YOU KNOW?

The skin eruption of shingles is considered one of the worst pains in medicine, rivaling corneal abrasions, chronic back pain, and the pain of labor and delivery. Shingles occurs in more than five hundred thousand people a year in the United States.

THINGS TO DO

Because there is little that can be done to alleviate the pain of shingles, the best way to avoid it is to get the shingles vaccine. Although people who have received the chickenpox vaccine can

(*continued on next page*)

(continued from previous page)

still get shingles, the disease is far more mild and less severe than episodes of shingles that result from reactivation of a natural chickenpox infection.

What Are the Symptoms of Shingles?

Shingles causes an intense, painful skin eruption with blisters on one side of the face or body. Before the rash appears, people often experience pain, itching, or tingling in the area where the rash ultimately develops. The rash typically scabs over in seven to ten days, but the pain of shingles, called post-herpetic neuralgia (PHN), can last for months and sometimes years. The scabs can also affect the area around the eye, causing difficulty with vision.

DID YOU KNOW?

The observation that chickenpox and shingles were caused by the same virus was first made in 1892.

ONE PERSON'S STORY

The inventor of nine of the fifteen vaccines currently given to infants and young children, Dr. Maurice Hilleman, suffered shingles toward the end of his life. Ironic given that he helped to develop the chickenpox vaccine.

SHINGLES: THE VACCINE

What Is the Shingles Vaccine?

The first shingles vaccine, Zostavax, was licensed in 2006. The vaccine was exactly the same as the chickenpox vaccine given to children, except that the dose was fourteen times greater.

Zostavax was later replaced by a different shingles vaccine, Shingrix, which was licensed in 2017. Unlike Zostavax, which consisted of live, weakened chickenpox virus, Shingrix contains only one viral protein, called glycoprotein E. This protein is responsible for attaching chickenpox virus to cells, so antibodies directed against glycoprotein E interfere with viral attachment to cells. More importantly, however, Shingrix is a powerful inducer of T cells, which are cells of the immune system responsible for killing virus-infected cells. This is critical in preventing shingles because when the chickenpox virus reactivates in one of the nerve roots of the central nervous system, it travels from cell to cell along a nerve path.

In addition to glycoprotein E, Shingrix contains two powerful adjuvants. One is called monophosphoryl lipid A (MPLA) and the other is a saponin (a soap) called QS-21 made from the bark of a tree found in Chile. A tribute to the power of these adjuvants is that Shingrix is the first vaccine in history in which a single protein induces a better protective response than a live, weakened virus (Zostavax). For that reason, the Centers for Disease Control and Prevention (CDC) expressed a preference for Shingrix over Zostavax. Indeed, Shingrix was recommended even for those who had already received Zostavax.

Who Should Get the Shingles Vaccine?

Shingles vaccine is recommended for anyone over fifty years of age. The vaccine is administered in two doses separated by two to six months. Some adults nineteen years of age and older with weakened immune systems because of disease or medical treatment should also receive two doses of Shingrix. If you're not sure whether your condition puts you in this category, talk with your health care provider.

Who Should Avoid or Delay Getting the Shingles Vaccine?

People who have a known allergy to any component of the shingles vaccine should avoid it. Similarly, anyone who has had a severe allergic reaction to the first dose of Shingrix should not get the second dose. People with moderate or severe illness, those who are pregnant, and those with a current case of shingles should delay vaccination.

Does the Shingles Vaccine Work?

The shingles vaccine protects more than 95 of 100 people, including those over seventy-five years of age.

What Are the Side Effects of the Shingles Vaccine?

Shingrix has a difficult side effect profile. More than half of vaccine recipients will develop systemic symptoms, such as muscle aches, fatigue, headache, shivering, fever, and intestinal symptoms. More than 75 of 100 vaccine recipients will develop pain, redness, and swelling at the injection site. In about 10 of 100 vaccine recipients, these symptoms can be severe enough to interfere with daily activities, like missing a day of work. While these side effects can be unwelcome, they are not long-lived, nor do they cause permanent harm. However, shingles disease can affect one's life for months or even permanently, and the pain associated with shingles can be so severe as to cause depression, anxiety, loss of ability to care for oneself, and suicidal thoughts.

DID YOU KNOW?

As we age, our immune system also ages, becoming somewhat less effective at preventing infections and responding to vaccines. The shingles vaccine is remarkable in that it is highly effective in those quite advanced in age. Probably no other vaccine is as effective in this age group.

Why Get the Shingles Vaccine?

1. *The pain of shingles can be long-lasting and life altering.* Anyone who has experienced the intense, unremitting pain of

shingles will tell you that they would have done anything to avoid it.

2. *About one in four people will experience shingles in their lifetime.* The risk increases after fifty years of age and becomes even more likely as people age, affecting up to one in two older adults.

3. *The shingles vaccine is safe and highly effective in all older age groups.* Although the side effects can cause a couple days of discomfort, the pain of shingles, which is far more intense and far more debilitating, can last for months or years.

SHINGLES: OTHER THINGS YOU MIGHT HAVE WONDERED ABOUT

Likelihood of Historical Chickenpox Exposure

Some people might not remember whether they've had chickenpox and therefore they may be unsure whether they're at risk for shingles. But chickenpox was common before the chickenpox vaccine was first licensed for all children in 1995. All people over the age of fifty years were born before 1995, so it is likely that they had chickenpox even if they don't remember.

Is Shingles Contagious?

Because shingles is a reactivation of a virus living in the affected person's cells, an affected person can't give someone else shingles. However, it is possible that people who have never had chickenpox can catch the virus from someone with shingles. This is most often a concern for infants younger than one year of age since they will not have had the vaccine yet. To prevent chickenpox infections, those with shingles should keep susceptible people away from the rash because it is contact with the lesions or liquid from them that can cause a chickenpox infection. If the rash has not yet developed, if it has crusted, or if it has healed (even if the pain lingers), a person with shingles cannot spread the virus to a susceptible person.

Can a Person Spread the Virus After Getting Vaccinated?

No. Shingrix contains only a single protein from the virus, so no whole virus is present, which means that people can't spread the virus after vaccination. The older shingles vaccine (Zostavax) contained live, weakened virus, so people could spread the virus to others who were not immune to chickenpox. Zostavax is no longer available in the United States.

Shingles: Additional Resources

ONLINE INFORMATION

"Do I Need to Avoid Being Around Infants After Getting a Shingles Vaccine?": https://www.chop.edu/centers-programs/vaccine-education -center/video/do-i-need-avoid-being-around-infants-after-shingles -vaccine

"A Look at Each Vaccine: Shingles Vaccine": https://www.chop.edu /centers-programs/vaccine-education-center/vaccine-details/shingles -vaccine

"Shingles": https://media.chop.edu/data/files/pdfs/shingles-disease -infographic.pdf

"Shingles Vaccine": https://www.voicesforvaccines.org/vaccine-information /shingles/

"Shingles: What You Should Know": https://media.chop.edu/data /files/pdfs/vaccine-education-center-shingles.pdf

"Shingles (Zoster)": https://www.vaccineinformation.org/diseases /shingles/

"The Stages of Viral Infection: How HPV and Shingles Play a Long Game": https://www.chop.edu/video/stages-viral-infection-how -hpv-and-shingles-play-long-game

"Talking About Vaccines with Dr. Paul Offit: News Briefs – January 2018 – New Shingles Vaccine Changes Recommendation for Adults": https://www.chop.edu/video/talking-about-vaccines-dr-paul -offit-news-briefs-january-2018-new-shingles-vaccine-changes

PHOTOS

"Shingles (zoster) Photos": https://www.vaccineinformation.org /photos/shingles/

PERSONAL EXPERIENCES

"Unprotected People Stories: Zoster (Shingles)": https://www.immunize
    .org/clinical/vaccine-confidence/unprotected-people/topic
    /zoster-shingles/

"Parents PACK Personal Stories – Shingles": https://www.chop.edu
    /centers-programs/parents-pack/personal-stories/shingles

"Story Gallery": https://www.shotbyshot.org/story-gallery/ (search
    "shingles")

MPOX

MPOX: THE DISEASE

The first case of monkeypox, now called mpox, appeared in the United States on May 17, 2022, in Boston, Massachusetts. Soon, the virus spread to all fifty states, causing more than thirty thousand cases of illness and thirty-eight deaths. On August 14, 2022, the United States declared a public health emergency, with more than four hundred cases being reported every day. With the availability of vaccines and antiviral drugs, the mpox epidemic declined dramatically.

What Is Mpox?

Mpox is a virus within the larger family of poxviruses. Many mammals have their own unique strains of poxvirus, for example, cowpox, horsepox, mousepox, swinepox, and human smallpox.

DID YOU KNOW?

Humankind's first vaccine was the smallpox vaccine, created by a British doctor named Edward Jenner. Jenner noticed that women who milked cows with blisters on their udders developed similar blisters on their hands and wrists. When smallpox swept across the English countryside every few years, milkmaids would often be spared the infection. Jenner reasoned that the milkmaids didn't get infected with smallpox because they had been previously infected with what we now know as cowpox. Cowpox didn't cause severe disease in people, but human smallpox did. The initial smallpox vaccine was cowpox.

ONE PERSON'S STORY

"All the unanswered questions took a toll on my mental health. I'd never been hospitalized before and the uncertainty around the disease was stressful. I was on heavy pain killers, on antibiotics because of a secondary bacterial infection, and being fed through an intravenous drip. All I wanted was for the pain to go away. . . . Even now, talking about the scars monkeypox could leave makes me emotional. I don't want to carry scars reminding me of this horrible month. I don't want to look at myself in the mirror and see this."

Source: "'We Always Think It's Not Going to Happen to Us' – A Sexual Health Worker's First-Hand Experience of Monkeypox." World Health Organization. July 15, 2022. https://www.who.int/europe/news/item/15 -07-2022-we-always-think-it-s-not-going-to-happen-to-us----a -sexual-health-worker-s-first-hand-experience-of-monkeypox.

What Are the Symptoms of Mpox?

People with mpox develop a rash that can be located on their hands, feet, chest, mouth, face, or genitals. The rash can appear anywhere between three and seventeen days after encountering someone infected with mpox. The rash is often painful and itchy.

Other symptoms of mpox include fever, chills, swollen lymph nodes, fatigue, muscle aches, headache, sore throat, congestion, and cough. The infection is spread from one person to another by close skin-to-skin contact with the affected area. Close skin-to-skin contact often occurs during a sexual encounter.

DID YOU KNOW?

Mpox can also be spread from animals to people.

MPOX: THE VACCINE

What Is the Mpox Vaccine?

The mpox vaccine, known as Jynneos, is composed of a poxvirus that is similar to cowpox; however, it has been cultured in the lab so that it cannot reproduce in human cells. The virus, called modified vaccinia Ankara (MVA), was used in other countries to vaccinate against smallpox in the last years before smallpox was eradicated, or eliminated from the world (1980). In other words, an immune response to one type of poxvirus (like cowpox) can protect against a poxvirus from a different species (like mpox or human smallpox). The vaccine virus isn't a killed virus (like the hepatitis A and polio vaccines). Nor is it a live, weakened virus that replicates in the vaccine recipient (like the measles and chickenpox vaccines). Rather, it is a live virus that cannot replicate when given to people. It is administered as a series of two doses with the second dose given at least four weeks after the first.

DID YOU KNOW?

Pregnant people can spread mpox virus to their fetus during pregnancy or to the newborn by close contact after birth.

DID YOU KNOW?

Jynneos is also used to protect against smallpox and other poxviruses. Although smallpox has been eradicated, some groups of people are at increased risk for exposure to poxviruses based on their work. This includes people who work on poxviruses or related research in labs. Some members of the U.S. military are also vaccinated against poxviruses.

Who Should Get the Mpox Vaccine?

The following groups are recommended to receive the mpox vaccine:

- Anyone with a known or suspected exposure to someone infected with mpox.
- Anyone who had sex within the past two weeks with a partner know to be diagnosed with mpox.
- Anyone who is gay or bisexual who has had more than one sexual partner within the past six months.
- Anyone with a sexual partner at increased risk of exposure to mpox, who works in settings that pose increased risk for exposure to infected individuals, or who works with mpox or other poxviruses in a laboratory setting.
- Children who have had skin-to-skin contact with someone who has mpox.

Who Should Avoid or Delay Getting the Mpox Vaccine?

People should not get a second dose of Jynneos if they had a severe allergic reaction to the first dose.

> **DID YOU KNOW?**
>
> The mpox vaccine can be administered either subcutaneously (under the skin) or intradermally (within the upper layer of the skin).

Does the Mpox Vaccine Work?

When the international mpox outbreak occurred in 2022, no formal, prospective, placebo-controlled studies of the Jynneos vaccine had been performed, but it was incumbent upon public health officials to use the data that were available to navigate the public health emergency. At the time, data from animals and immunologic data from people were available. In the latter studies, Jynneos had been compared to the smallpox vaccine and found to induce a similar immune response. Given that the smallpox vaccine had been found to be highly effective at preventing smallpox, it could reasonably be inferred that the mpox vaccine would also be highly effective at preventing mpox. So, the vaccine was recommended for those at greatest risk for mpox. However, officials also kept collecting data, and in mid-2023 the first data from a small study conducted by the New York State Department of Health confirmed their expectations. After receiving one dose, about 68 of 100 people were protected, and after the recommended two doses, about 88 or 89 of 100 people were protected. We can expect more data to emerge in the future as the vaccine continues to be used.

What Are the Side Effects of the Mpox Vaccine?

The most common side effects from the Jynneos vaccine are pain, redness, and itching at the injection site. Some people might also experience fever, headache, fatigue, nausea, chills, and muscle aches.

DID YOU KNOW?

Because of the smallpox vaccine, smallpox, a disease estimated to have killed more than five hundred million people, has been eliminated from the face of the earth.

Why Get the Mpox Vaccine?

1. *Mpox can cause a painful rash as well as a series of other symptoms; in a small number of cases, it can be fatal.* Beginning in 2022, an mpox epidemic swept across the United States, causing tens of thousands of cases and dozens of deaths. Not everyone was at risk, however. The disease occurred primarily following sexual contact with an infected person. But children and adults who

had close skin-to-skin, nonsexual contact with an infected person were also infected.

2. *The Jynneos vaccine is safe and effective.* The good news about the vaccine is that it works even if administered shortly *after* someone has been exposed to mpox. If a person finds out they were exposed, they should get vaccinated as soon as possible, ideally within four days of exposure. It is possible that even if vaccinated within two weeks of exposure, some protection will be afforded.

Mpox: Additional Resources

ONLINE INFORMATION

"Mpox": https://www.cdc.gov/poxvirus/mpox/index.html

"Mpox": https://www.vaccineinformation.org/diseases/mpox/

"Mpox (Monkeypox)": https://www.who.int/health-topics/monkeypox

PHOTOS

"Clinical Recognition": https://www.cdc.gov/poxvirus/mpox/clinicians/clinical-recognition.html

RESPIRATORY SYNCYTIAL VIRUS (RSV)

RSV: THE DISEASE

Respiratory syncytial virus (RSV) is one of several respiratory viruses that cause disease in the winter. Other winter respiratory viruses include influenza, parainfluenza, human metapneumovirus, and COVID-19. Collectively, these viruses cause hundreds of thousands of hospitalizations and tens of thousands of deaths every winter in the United States. In 2023, vaccines to prevent severe RSV infection in people sixty years of age and older were approved for use in the United States.

What Is RSV?

RSV is a common virus. The disease is particularly severe in infants in the first two months of life and in older adults.

> **DID YOU KNOW?**
>
> RSV was first found to be a cause of human disease in 1956. It has not been found to infect any types of animals.

What Are the Symptoms of RSV?

RSV can infect both the upper respiratory tract (i.e., the nose and throat) and the lower respiratory tract (i.e., the lungs). Symptoms of upper respiratory tract infection include runny nose, congestion, and sore throat. Symptoms of lower respiratory tract infection include cough, wheezing, increased sputum production, shortness of breath, difficulty breathing, and increased rate of breathing. Both upper and lower respiratory infections can cause fever, fatigue, body aches, headache, and decreased appetite. Severe infection of the lower respiratory tract (i.e., pneumonia) can cause a need for supplemental oxygen and occasionally mechanical ventilation in the intensive care unit.

DID YOU KNOW?

Most people have been infected with RSV by the time they are three years old. Mild infections can reoccur throughout life.

ONE PERSON'S STORY

"As someone who leads an active lifestyle—from kayaking to chasing my grandkids around—I am not one to easily be taken down. After having a persistent cough for more than a month, I knew something was wrong. I went to see my pulmonologist, but I left without a diagnosis. Instead, my doctor gave me an inhaler and recommended a few over-the-counter treatment options. . . . The coughing was so bad that I considered going to the hospital multiple times. My breathing was labored, my chest was tight, and overall, I felt extremely lousy and fatigued. I even had to sleep sitting up to avoid having a coughing fit. I used heat and steam to try to feel better, but nothing really helped—it felt like flu without the associated fever."

Source: "Susan's Story." National Foundation for Infectious Diseases. Accessed October 10, 2023, at https://www.nfid.org/resource/susans-story-rsv/.

RSV: THE VACCINE
What Is the RSV Vaccine?

Two RSV vaccines are available for people sixty years of age and older. One is made by Pfizer and the other by GSK. Both vaccines contain a protein located on the surface of the virus called the fusion protein. The fusion protein is responsible for attaching RSV to cells of the respiratory tract. Targeting a surface protein on the virus to prevent it from attaching to cells is the same strategy used to make the COVID-19 vaccines.

Vaccine-derived antibodies directed against the fusion protein prevent the virus from attaching to cells, thereby preventing infection.

The RSV vaccines are similar to the Novavax COVID-19 vaccine in that they deliver the protein directly, rather than having our cells generate the protein, like the mRNA or viral vector COVID-19 vaccines do. Pfizer's RSV vaccine does not contain an adjuvant. GSK's vaccine contains the same adjuvant used in Shingrix (i.e., monophosphoryl lipid A plus QS-21). These vaccines are given as a single shot in the fall to provide the greatest protection during the upcoming winter season.

In October 2023, Pfizer's RSV vaccine was approved for use in pregnant people between 32 and 36 weeks of gestation if their baby will be born during RSV season. This recommendation aims to protect the baby in the first few months of life when they are most susceptible to RSV.

DID YOU KNOW?

While RSV can infect people of any age, those over eighty years of age are thirty times more likely to be hospitalized than children.

DID YOU KNOW?

Of those hospitalized with RSV, more than 90 percent have at least one health problem that puts them at increased risk for severe disease. High-risk medical conditions include heart, lung, or kidney disease, diabetes, and immune-compromising conditions.

Who Should Get the RSV Vaccine?

Anyone sixty years of age and older may get a single dose in consultation with their health care provider.

Pregnant people likely to deliver during RSV season can get one dose of Pfizer's RSV vaccine between 32 and 36 weeks of gestation.

Who Should Avoid or Delay Getting the RSV Vaccine?
People who have had an allergic reaction to the shingles vaccine might also be allergic to the adjuvants in GSK's RSV vaccine. In which case, they should opt for the Pfizer RSV vaccine.

> **DID YOU KNOW?**
>
> Researchers had been trying to create an RSV vaccine for children and adults since the early 1960s without success. It took more than sixty years to make this vaccine.

Does the RSV Vaccine Work?
Both Pfizer's and GSK's RSV vaccines have been shown to be 85 to 95 percent effective at preventing severe illness during the first winter following vaccination. Each vaccine protects about 60 to 70 of 100 vaccinated people against mild disease several months after vaccination. The vaccines are also highly effective two years after vaccination. It remains to be seen whether efficacy against severe RSV infection holds up several years after inoculation. If not, the RSV vaccine might need to be given every few years. Unlike influenza, however, RSV does not evolve, so the vaccine will not need to be updated each year.

When Pfizer's vaccine was given to pregnant people between thirty-two and thirty-six weeks of pregnancy, their babies were less likely to be hospitalized or need medical attention if infected with RSV. The vaccine protected about 50 to 60 of 100 babies.

What Are the Side Effects of the RSV Vaccine?
The RSV vaccine causes pain at the injection site in about 10 of 100 recipients and swelling and redness at the site in less than

5 of 100 recipients. The incidence of fatigue, headache, muscle pain, and joint pain was no different between those who had been vaccinated and those who had received a placebo.

When given Pfizer's RSV vaccine, pregnant people experienced similar side effects to those experienced by older adults, such as injection site pain, headache, muscle pain, and nausea. However, one important side effect that occurred at a low rate, but still more frequently than in the placebo group, was preterm birth. Although this finding was not statistically significant, the CDC recommendations limited receipt of the RSV vaccine to between thirty-two and thirty-six weeks of gestation, rather than between twenty-four and thirty-six weeks as tested. Scientists and public health officials will carefully monitor whether receipt of the RSV vaccine is causally associated with preterm delivery as more doses of RSV vaccine are administered during pregnancy. If the association between vaccination and preterm delivery is supported by additional evidence, vaccine recommendations may be altered or use of the vaccine during pregnancy may be stopped. If you are pregnant and considering whether to receive the RSV vaccine, talk with your health care provider about the latest data related to these concerns.

Why Get the RSV Vaccine?

1. *RSV is a common cause of hospitalization and death in older adults.* Every year in the United States, RSV causes 3.4 million cases of illness, 1.7 million outpatient visits, about 150,000 hospitalizations, and 10,000 deaths in those sixty years of age and older.
2. *RSV vaccines are safe and effective for older adults.* We now have a vaccine to prevent the enormous burden of severe and occasionally fatal disease caused by RSV among older people. In two large clinical trials involving a total of about sixty thousand participants, the vaccine has been shown to be safe and effective.
3. *RSV vaccination during pregnancy can protect new babies from RSV during their most vulnerable period.* When RSV vaccine is

given between thirty-two and thirty-six weeks of gestation in anticipation of delivery during RSV season, maternal RSV antibodies are passed to the unborn baby so that they are protected in the weeks and months after birth.

RSV: Additional Resources

ONLINE INFORMATION

"Closing the Gap: Disparities and Respiratory Syncytial Virus (RSV)": https://www.youtube.com/watch?v=aeoQCyjFLQU

"A Look at Each Vaccine: Respiratory Syncytial Virus (RSV) Vaccine and Monoclonal Antibody": https://www.chop.edu/centers-programs /vaccine-education-center/vaccine-details/rsv-vaccine-monoclonal -antibody

"Respiratory Syncytial Virus Infection (RSV)": https://www.cdc.gov /rsv/index.html

"Respiratory Syncytial Virus (RSV)": https://www.nfid.org/infectious -disease/rsv/

"RSV: A Virus You Should Know": https://www.youtube.com/watch?v =3eLlotbY-z4

Vaccines and Related Biological Products Advisory Committee February 28–March 1, 2023, Meeting Announcement": https://www.fda .gov/advisory-committees/advisory-committee-calendar/vaccines -and-related-biological-products-advisory-committee-february -28-march-1-2023-meeting#event-materials (meeting presentation materials)

THE VACCINE SCHEDULE

THE VACCINE SCHEDULE

Birth

The first dose of hepatitis B vaccine is given at birth.

Two Months

If your child visits the doctor at one month of age, the second dose of hepatitis B vaccine may be given. However, most doctors give the second dose at the two-month visit.

Also given at the two-month visit are the first doses of the rotavirus; diphtheria, tetanus, and pertussis (DTaP); *Haemophilus influenzae* type b (Hib); pneumococcal; and polio vaccines.

To reduce the number of shots, some vaccines are combined. To find out more, see the "Combination Vaccines" section at the end of this chapter.

Four Months

The second doses of rotavirus, DTaP, Hib, pneumococcal, and polio vaccines are typically given at the four-month visit.

To reduce the number of shots, some vaccines are combined. To find out more, see the "Combination Vaccines" section at the end of this chapter.

Six Months

The third dose of hepatitis B vaccine is given between six and eighteen months of age. Many doctors give it at the six-month visit.

If the rotavirus vaccine, RotaTeq, was administered for either or both of the first two doses, a third dose should be given at six months of age.

Similarly, if any brand of the Hib vaccine—except the one known as PedvaxHIB—was given, the child should get a third dose at six months of age.

Also given at the six-month visit are the third doses of the DTaP and pneumococcal vaccines. The third dose of the polio vaccine can be given any time between six and eighteen months of age.

The first dose of COVID-19 vaccine is also recommended at six months of age. The number of doses and timing depend on which brand of vaccine is administered. It is recommended to use the same brand for all doses whenever possible.

To reduce the number of shots, some vaccines are combined. To find out more, see the "Combination Vaccines" section at the end of this chapter.

COVID-19 Vaccine

Infants are recommended to get COVID-19 vaccine beginning at six months of age. Anyone older than six months of age who remains unvaccinated against COVID-19 should also consider getting the vaccine as recommended for their age and health situation, regardless of whether they have had a previous COVID-19 infection. Studies have indicated that hybrid immunity, that is, immunity resulting from both infection and vaccination, affords the most robust protection.

The Centers for Disease Control and Prevention (CDC) currently recommends an annual COVID-19 vaccine for almost everyone; however, four specific groups of people are most likely to benefit:

- Individuals aged sixty-five years and older
- Individuals with health conditions that increase their risk of severe disease, particularly, diabetes, obesity, and chronic conditions of the heart, lungs, liver, or kidneys
- Individuals who are immune compromised either because of health conditions or medical treatments
- Pregnant people

Annual Influenza Vaccine

The influenza vaccine is recommended yearly starting at six months of age. The first time a child receives it, two doses separated by at least one month are required.

Influenza shots can be given safely with any other vaccine. Because different types are given as a shot, some brands can be administered to anyone older than six months of age, whereas other brands are limited to adults of certain ages.

The nasal-spray version can be given at the same time as any other vaccine except another nasal-spray vaccine (although currently, no other nasal-spray vaccines are approved for use in the United States). Because the nasal-spray version contains live, weakened influenza viruses, if it is not given at the same time as other vaccines containing live, weakened viruses (e.g., chickenpox or MMR), the vaccines must be separated by one month from each other. The nasal-spray vaccine should not be given to children less than two years old.

Influenza vaccines are not available in combination with other vaccines.

Find out more about the different types of influenza vaccine and which age groups they can be used by in the "Influenza" section of the "Vaccines in the First Year of Life" chapter.

Twelve to Eighteen Months

The third and final dose of hepatitis B vaccine may be given any time between six and eighteen months of age.

The third or fourth dose of Hib vaccine (depending on brand) and the fourth dose of pneumococcal vaccine are given between twelve and fifteen months, and the fourth dose of DTaP vaccine is given between fifteen and eighteen months.

The third dose of polio vaccine may be given any time between six and eighteen months.

The first doses of measles, mumps, and rubella (MMR) and chickenpox vaccines are given between twelve and fifteen months.

The first and second doses of hepatitis A vaccine are given between twelve and twenty-three months.

If a child has not received all recommended doses of COVID-19 vaccine, they should start or continue that vaccine during these months.

To reduce the number of shots, some vaccines are combined. To find out more, see the "Combination Vaccines" section at the end of this chapter.

Eighteen Months to Four Years

Between eighteen months and four years of age, children should get an annual influenza vaccine and catch up on any recommended vaccine doses they did not complete during their first eighteen months of life.

Four to Six Years

The next series of routine vaccines are recommended between four and six years of age as children prepare to start school. Vaccine doses recommended during this period include the fifth dose of DTaP vaccine, second doses of MMR and chickenpox vaccines, and the fourth dose of polio vaccine. Children should also receive an annual influenza vaccine throughout this period, and they should catch up on any doses of recommended vaccines not yet received.

To reduce the number of shots, some vaccines are combined. To find out more, see the "Combination Vaccines" section at the end of this chapter.

Seven to Ten Years

If children are up to date on recommended vaccines, they will typically not require many doses during this period. However, you should be aware of a few vaccines during these years:

- Influenza vaccine is recommended annually; previous vaccination does not guarantee protection in subsequent years because of how quickly the virus changes.
- Human papillomavirus (HPV) vaccine can be administered beginning at nine years of age. While this vaccine is typically recommended starting at eleven years of age, health care providers and parents may opt for earlier dosing for a few reasons. First, children will need fewer vaccines at eleven years of age. Second, as children get older, their schedules get busier, and this vaccine requires at least two doses separated by six to twelve months. Finally, the vaccine has been shown to be most effective at younger ages (before fifteen years of age), and protection has been demonstrated to be long-lasting, so getting children protected sooner often makes sense to parents and providers.
- Dengue vaccine is recommended for those nine to sixteen years of age who live in areas where dengue is endemic *and* have proof of previous dengue infection. Check with your child's health care provider if you're uncertain about whether your child needs this vaccine. Currently, the areas included in this recommendation are Puerto Rico, American Samoa, U.S. Virgin Islands, Federated States of Micronesia, Republic of the Marshall Islands, and Republic of Palau; however, this could change over time, so a local health care provider or public health official will be your best source of information. To find out more about dengue and the vaccine,

see the "Dengue" section of the "Vaccines for 7- to 18-year-olds" chapter.

Eleven to Twelve Years

Tdap, meningococcal, and HPV vaccines are recommended for adolescents. Tdap and meningococcal vaccines require a single dose at this age. HPV vaccines require two or three doses, depending on the age at which vaccination occurs. Those younger than fifteen years of age require two doses separated by six to twelve months, whereas those fifteen years of age and older require three doses. The second dose should be administered one to two months after the first dose and the third dose at least six months after the first dose.

Dengue vaccine may be recommended during this period if an adolescent did not receive it at an earlier age and if they qualify for it because of where they live and their history of exposure to the virus. Find out more in the "Dengue" section of the "Vaccines for 7- to 18-year-olds" chapter.

Adolescents should also receive an annual influenza vaccine, and they should catch up on any missed vaccine doses.

The vaccines given at this age are not available in combination.

Thirteen to Eighteen Years

In addition to an annual influenza vaccine and any "catch-up" doses if they have fallen behind, a teen may need a few other vaccines during this period:

- An additional dose or doses of meningococcal vaccine may be needed, depending on which meningococcal vaccine they received previously. For example, unless a teen is at increased risk of meningococcal disease because of a health condition, many parents are unaware that a meningococcal B vaccine is available. The MenB vaccine is recommended for those sixteen to twenty-three years of age who are not at increased risk following a discussion between the teen's parents and health care provider. It is administered as two doses separated by either one month or six months, depending on which brand of vaccine is given. See the "Meningococcus" section of the "Vaccines for 7- to 18-year-olds" chapter for more information about this vaccine.

- Dengue vaccine may be recommended for teens during this period if they did not receive it at an earlier age and if they qualify for it because of where they live and their history of exposure to the virus. Find out more in the "Dengue" section of the "Vaccines for 7- to 18-year-olds" chapter.

Nineteen to Forty-Nine Years

Adults in this age group should be immune to diseases like measles, mumps, rubella, and chickenpox. Immunity is most often from vaccination, but in some cases, a history of disease is sufficient. Check with your health care provider if you have questions about your situation. For adults who need to be vaccinated for protection against these diseases, one or two doses are usually needed, depending on the situation. If two doses are needed, in most cases they should be separated by at least four weeks. Your health care provider will determine your dosing needs based on the adult immunization schedule.

This group of adults should also be up to date on recommended vaccines that may have been missed at an earlier age, such as hepatitis B vaccine (two to four doses). And they should get vaccines recommended on routine schedules, such as influenza and COVID-19 vaccines (one dose every year) and Tdap or Td (one dose every ten years). In some cases, Tdap or Td is recommended during a shorter interval, such as following a wound or during pregnancy.

Those aged nineteen to twenty-six years are recommended to get the HPV vaccine if they have not yet received it, and those between twenty-seven and forty-five years of age can decide in consultation with their health care provider whether they might benefit from receiving HPV vaccine. For someone who has never been vaccinated against HPV, three doses are recommended, with the second dose given one to two months after the first dose and the third dose given at least six months after the first dose. For someone who has received some but not all recommended doses of HPV vaccine, the number and timing of doses will depend on their previous doses.

Adults who would like to be protected against hepatitis A can get that vaccine, and it is worth considering because hepatitis A infections do not result only from international travel. Hepatitis A vaccine typically requires two doses separated by at least six months; however, if an individual gets the combination vaccine called Twinrix, they will need three doses (see the "Combination Vaccines" section of this chapter for more details).

Some adults may be recommended to get other vaccines, depending on whether they have certain health conditions. Vaccines recommended for certain groups include those for pneumococcus, meningococcus, Hib, and shingles. Talk with your health care provider if you're uncertain whether you are recommended to get any of these vaccines. Your health care provider can also provide information about the number of doses and relative timing of each, as some variability exists depending on why a person is recommended to get a particular vaccine.

Fifty Years and Older

As adults get older, they may be recommended to get vaccines that were not previously recommended simply because of their age:

- Beginning at fifty years of age, two doses of shingles vaccine separated by two to six months are recommended. People older than fifty years of age who have not received two doses of this vaccine are also recommended to get it.
- Beginning at sixty years of age, adults are recommended to receive the respiratory syncytial virus (RSV) vaccine after discussion with their health care provider about the relative risks and benefits of vaccination.
- Beginning at sixty-five years of age, adults who were not previously vaccinated against pneumococcus or for whom vaccination

history is unknown should get one or two doses, depending on which pneumococcal vaccine they will be getting. Adults who have previously received pneumococcal vaccine—and know which one they received—typically need only one dose, but which vaccine they need will depend on their existing vaccination history.

Adults fifty years of age and older should also follow the dosing recommendations for influenza, COVID-19 and Tdap or Td vaccines. If they have not previously been vaccinated against hepatitis A and hepatitis B, they can get these vaccines. The hepatitis A vaccine is given in two doses separated by at least six months, and the hepatitis B vaccine is typically given in two or three doses, depending on which vaccine is used.

Some adults may require additional vaccines, depending on their age, risk factors, and vaccination history. Talk with your health care provider about your situation, or check out the CDC's Adult Vaccine Assessment Tool: https://www2.cdc.gov /nip/adultimmsched/.

THINGS TO DO

For the most up-to-date immunization schedules, consult the CDC website:

- Birth to six years: https://www.cdc.gov/vaccines/schedules /easy-to-read/child-easyread.html
- Seven to eighteen years: https://www.cdc.gov/vaccines /schedules/easy-to-read/adolescent-easyread.html
- Nineteen years and older: https://www.cdc.gov/vaccines /adults/index.html

WHY THIS SCHEDULE?

Several groups determine the U.S. vaccine schedules. Each group is composed of committees of experts who review results from

vaccine trials. Trial data typically include the ages of trial participants, how many doses were required to afford protection, the
presence of side effects, and the safety and efficacy of the vaccine when given with other vaccines typically administered at
the same time (such studies are called concomitant-use studies).

Experts also study how the disease affects individuals who
have it, which groups of people get it, how many people it affects
each year, and when and where the disease is occurring. All this
information determines which vaccines are added to the schedule, when, for whom, and the number of doses needed.

Once a vaccine has been added to the schedule, these groups
continue to monitor both the disease and the vaccine. They want
to make sure that the vaccine is working and is safe and that
disease is decreasing. Sometimes the schedule will be adjusted
to better use the vaccine by changing recommendations, such as
who should get the vaccine or the number of doses needed.

The groups that review and approve data related to the child-
hood and adolescent schedule include the CDC, American
Academy of Pediatrics, American Academy of Family Physicians
(AAFP), American College of Obstetricians and Gynecologists
(ACOG), American College of Nurse-Midwives (ACNM),
American Academy of Physician Associates (AAPA), and National
Association of Pediatric Nurse Practitioners.

The groups that review and approve data related to the adult
schedule include the CDC, AAFP, ACOG, ACNM, AAPA,
American College of Physicians, American Pharmacists Association, and Society for Healthcare Epidemiology of America.

CHANGES TO THE SCHEDULE

The vaccine schedules are updated annually; however, changes
can occur throughout the year as new vaccines become available
or as changes are deemed necessary. Changes can be made for
several reasons.

A new vaccine becomes available. A new vaccine can be the first
of its kind or another version of an existing vaccine. For example,

during late 2021 and early 2022, several new COVID-19 vaccines became available. Likewise, in 2022 a new version of the MMR vaccine, called Priorix, became available. This vaccine is similar to the existing MMR vaccine, called MMR II; however, it's made by another company, which better ensures a continued supply for babies in the United States.

Extra doses of a vaccine are needed. When a vaccine is first added to the schedule, many people are spreading the infection. As vaccine use increases, fewer people spread disease, so there are fewer opportunities for people to be exposed and "remind" their immune system about the pathogen. Although people don't realize they're being exposed to the pathogen (because the vaccine has worked to protect them from illness), such exposures strengthen their immune response. However, sometimes a point is reached when there's so little community transmission that another dose of vaccine becomes necessary to maintain a robust immunologic memory. In part, this occurred when second doses of the MMR and chickenpox vaccines were added to the schedule for four- to six-year-olds.

Additional groups of people are recommended to get the vaccine. When a new vaccine is added to the schedule, it is sometimes recommended only for certain people. This can happen for a few reasons, such as a need to focus on the highest-risk groups, a limited initial supply of the vaccine, or the availability of data only in certain groups. For example, the hepatitis A vaccine was originally recommended for children in geographic regions where the rates of disease were high, but as the vaccine was used in those regions, other areas emerged as the most common sites of hepatitis A disease. So, the schedule was changed to include all children between twelve and twenty-three months of age. More recently, because of outbreaks among subpopulations of high-risk adults, the recommendations changed again to include older children and teens who had not previously been vaccinated (as part of what's called a catch-up campaign), specific groups of high-risk adults, and anyone who wants to be protected against hepatitis A.

The influenza vaccine is an example of a vaccine recommended to gradually increasing numbers of people because originally there was not enough vaccine to go around even though everyone is at some risk of severe influenza infection. As manufacturers were able to increase their production and as more types of influenza vaccine became available, greater numbers of people were recommended to get the vaccine. By the 2010–2011 influenza season, everyone older than six months of age was recommended to get vaccinated against influenza.

The HPV vaccine is an example of expanding recommendations based on new data for certain groups. When the vaccine was first made available, it had been tested only in girls and young women; however, after the manufacturer was able to test it in boys and young men, the recommendation was expanded to include all adolescents and teens. This expanded recommendation now allows males to be protected from anal, genital, and oral warts and cancers and to decrease the spread of this virus.

There is a vaccine shortage. If a vaccine is in short supply, the schedule may be changed so that the maximum number of children can be protected. For example, in December 2007, a shortage of the Hib vaccine required that health care providers withhold the last dose of the vaccine (typically given between twelve and fifteen months of age) until supplies could be replenished. Unfortunately, this problem might have led to increases in the amount of Hib bacteria circulating in the community and may have contributed to outbreaks in 2008.

THE CATCH-UP SCHEDULE

People may miss doses of vaccines because of illness, vaccine shortages, or changes to the schedule. As a result, each year, in addition to the regular immunization schedule for children and adolescents, a catch-up schedule is published to aid health care providers and families in determining a child's vaccine needs. While an adult "catch-up" table is not published, the adult immunization schedule includes a series of notes to help health care providers and families determine an adult's vaccine needs.

THINGS TO DO

Because the immunization schedule can change and individuals can miss doses for a variety of reasons, it's a good practice to ask whether you need any vaccines at every medical appointment. And if you're diagnosed with a new chronic condition, it's helpful to ask whether the condition warrants any special approach to vaccinations. In some cases, a condition increases the number of vaccines an individual needs, but in other cases, the condition or a medication taken for its treatment may limit a person's ability to get certain vaccines.

COMBINATION VACCINES

To reduce the number of shots per visit for infants and young children, some vaccines have been combined. Your health care provider's office is likely to use one or more of these combination vaccines; however, it's important to realize that some combinations contain different mixtures of vaccines and are approved for different age groups. The most important considerations for parents of young children when it comes to combination vaccines are that they have been tested for the ages at which they are approved to be used and that by combining vaccines, the number of shots a child will get at a single visit and the opportunity for vaccine administration mistakes both decrease. Combination vaccines have been shown to be just as safe and effective as the individual vaccines given at the same visit with a few exceptions, which are noted in the following list.

Combination vaccines currently available in the United States include:

- *Kinrix* and *Quadracel* are combination vaccines made by different manufacturers. Both contain diphtheria, tetanus, pertussis, and inactivated polio vaccines, and both are administered to children between four and six years of age. Kinrix causes pain, redness, and swelling at the injection site in about four additional children of 100 when compared with those who receive separate vaccines.

- *Pediarix* contains diphtheria, tetanus, pertussis, inactivated polio, and hepatitis B vaccines. This vaccine can be given to children between six weeks and six years of age. Pediarix causes redness or swelling at the injection site in about 7 of 100 more infants compared with those who receive separate vaccines. Likewise, about 8 of 100 additional infants will have fever compared with those who receive individual doses.
- *Pentacel* contains diphtheria, tetanus, pertussis, inactivated polio, and Hib vaccines. This vaccine can be given to children between six weeks and four years of age.
- *Vaxelis* contains diphtheria, tetanus, pertussis, inactivated polio, Hib, and hepatitis B vaccines. This vaccine can be given to children between six weeks and four years of age. It's generally used only for infants at the two-month, four-month, and six-month vaccine visits. About 13 more babies of every 100 who get this vaccine will experience a fever compared with 100 who get Pentacel and hepatitis B vaccines. However, the rates of visits to the doctor's office or emergency department due to fever do not differ between the two groups.
- *ProQuad* contains measles, mumps, rubella, and chickenpox vaccines. This vaccine, commonly referred to as MMRV, can be given to children between twelve months and twelve years of age. The vaccine causes a fever of 102°F or higher in about six out of 100 additional children compared with those given the vaccines separately. An additional one of 100 children may get a measles-like rash. Importantly, after the first dose of ProQuad, an additional one of every 2,600 children is likely to have seizure associated with fever in the first one to two weeks after getting the vaccine compared with children who receive the two vaccines separately at the same visit. For this reason, the CDC suggests that parents and health care providers discuss the relative risks and benefits

of getting the combined or separate versions. While parents and health care providers have the option of giving the combined version, the CDC has expressed a preference for using the two separate vaccines (MMR and chickenpox) for the first dose at twelve months of age or, if the child is behind, any first dose administered before four years of age. However, because the increased risk of fever-related seizures is not associated with the second dose or ages older than four years, any child getting their second dose (even if before the age of four) or getting their first dose after the age of four can get MMRV. In these scenarios, the CDC expresses a preference for using the combination vaccine since it requires one less shot.

- *Twinrix* contains hepatitis A and hepatitis B vaccines. It is approved for those eighteen years of age and older.

APPENDIXES

VACCINE RECORDS AND REGISTRIES

It's important to keep track of which vaccines the members of your family have received and when. You will need this information throughout life, and it's often easier when you know where it is and can access it quickly. Children and young adults often need their immunization records when registering for schools, camps, and colleges. In addition, individuals of any age may be required to show an immunization record to potential employers, for international travel, or for medical purposes. The easiest way to keep track of this information is to keep all the dates in a single place, such as on a paper—or electronic—immunization record.

In this section you will find photocopy-ready record pages that can be updated following receipt of vaccinations, making it easy to know which vaccines each family member has received and when. This is especially useful when adding or switching doctors.

In some cases, medical offices are part of statewide or local immunization registries. Registries are computer-based applications that track immunizations and sometimes other health-related information, such as vision and lead screenings. Registries are secure and confidential, and they allow for better health care in several ways. First, because the records are in a computer database, the information is centralized, allowing health care providers from multiple practices to access them with a patient's permission (or in the case of a child, their parent or caregiver's permission). For example, if you switch doctors because you moved, a registry can allow the new doctor to get your family's immunization records. Or, if your child sees a pediatrician and a specialist, both can consult the registry to determine whether immunizations are needed. Second, many registries are set up to automatically indicate when a vaccine is needed, so a busy provider will be alerted that vaccines are due even if you are at the doctor's office for another reason. Many offices no longer send reminders about immunizations, so registries provide a good way to be sure each patient is up to date. Third, registries have been shown to reduce the number of "extra" doses of vaccine that are given. In many cases, if a doctor isn't sure whether a patient has had a vaccine, they will recommend getting it anyway. The extra dose is not harmful, and the provider likely wants to err on the side of caution by making sure the patient is protected. By keeping the information in the registry and eliminating questions about previous doses, health care costs and the number of shots given to a patient can be reduced.

If your doctor's office is part of a registry or if they have an electronic medical record system, you may get copies showing which vaccines were administered at each visit. These records should be saved, but you may still choose to transfer the information onto a comprehensive record page so that you have all the information in one place. In some cases, you may be able to download certain medical information, such as previous immunizations; however, it is important to remember to do this periodically or before changing health care providers in case you lose access (or your password).

DID YOU KNOW?

Following Hurricane Katrina in September 2005, the importance of registries became apparent as many displaced families lost their health records. This was a problem for emergency personnel trying to determine who needed vaccines to prevent potential outbreaks that often occur following a natural disaster. Registries also helped with school registration for displaced children. For those children already in registries, the information was invaluable.

TEMPLATES FOR KEEPING TRACK OF VACCINES

RECORD OF IMMUNIZATIONS FOR _____ *DATE OF BIRTH* _____

VACCINE	NUMBER OF DOSES (BIRTH–6 YEARS)					
	1	2	3	4	5	6
Hepatitis B						
Rotavirus						
Diphtheria, tetanus, and pertussis						
Haemophilus influenzae type b						
Pneumococcus						
Polio						
Influenza						
Measles, mumps, and rubella						
Varicella (chickenpox)						
Hepatitis A						
COVID-19						
Other						

NOTES _____

_____

_____

_____

RECORD OF IMMUNIZATIONS FOR _____ DATE OF BIRTH _____

VACCINE	NUMBER OF DOSES (7–18 YEARS)					
	1	2	3	4	5	6
Diphtheria, tetanus, and pertussis						
Human papillomavirus (HPV)						
Meningococcal						
Influenza						
Dengue						
Other						
Other						
Other						
Other						
Other						
Other						

NOTES _____

_____

_____

RECORD OF IMMUNIZATIONS FOR _____ DATE OF BIRTH _____

VACCINE	NUMBER OF DOSES (19 YEARS AND OLDER)					
	1	2	3	4	5	6
Diphtheria, tetanus, and pertussis						
Human papillomavirus (HPV)						
Hepatitis B						
Pneumococcal						
Shingles						
COVID-19						
Influenza						
Hepatitis A						
Mpox						
Respiratory syncytial virus (RSV)						
Other						
Other						

NOTES_____

_____

_____

_____

SELECTED RESOURCES

REFERENCE BOOKS

Centers for Disease Control and Prevention. *CDC Yellow Book 2024*. New York: Oxford University Press, 2024.

Centers for Disease Control and Prevention. *Epidemiology and Prevention of Vaccine-Preventable Diseases*, 14th ed. Washington, DC: Public Health Foundation, 2021.

Feemster, Kristen A. *Vaccines: What Everyone Needs to Know*. New York: Oxford University Press, 2018.

Marshall, Gary S. *The Vaccine Handbook: A Practical Guide for Clinicians*, 7th ed. West Islip, NY: Professional Communications, 2018.

Orenstein, Walter A., Paul A. Offit, Kathryn M. Edwards, and Stanley A. Plotkin, eds. *Plotkin's Vaccines*, 8th ed. London: Elsevier, 2024.

MEDICAL NARRATIVES

Barry, John M. *The Great Influenza: The Story of the Deadliest Pandemic in History*. New York: Penguin, 2004.

Foege, William H. *House on Fire: The Fight to Eradicate Smallpox*. Berkeley: University of California Press, 2011.

Mnookin, Seth. *The Panic Virus: A True Story of Medicine, Science, and Fear*. New York: Simon & Schuster, 2011.

Offit, Paul A. *Autism's False Prophets: Bad Science, Risky Medicine, and the Search for a Cure*. New York: Columbia University Press, 2010.

——. *Bad Advice: Or Why Celebrities, Politicians, and Activists Aren't Your Best Source of Health Information*. New York: Columbia University Press, 2018.

——. *Bad Faith: When Religious Belief Undermines Modern Medicine*. New York: Basic Books, 2015.

——. *The Cutter Incident: How America's First Polio Vaccine Led to the Growing Vaccine Crisis*. New Haven, CT: Yale University Press, 2005.

——. *Deadly Choices: How the Anti-vaccine Movement Threatens Us All*. New York: Basic Books, 2012.

——. *Do You Believe in Magic? Vitamins, Supplements, and All Things Natural: A Look Behind the Curtain*. New York: HarperCollins, 2013.

——. *Overkill: When Modern Medicine Goes Too Far*. New York: HarperCollins, 2020.

——. *Pandora's Lab: Seven Stories of Science Gone Wrong*. Washington, DC: National Geographic, 2017.

——. *Tell Me When It's Over: An Insider's Guide to Deciphering COVID Myths and Navigating Our Post-Pandemic World*. New York: National Geographic, 2024.

——. *Vaccinated: One Man's Quest to Defeat the World's Deadliest Diseases*. New York: Smithsonian, 2007.

——. *You Bet Your Life: From Blood Transfusions to Mass Vaccination, the Long and Risky History of Medical Innovation*. New York: Basic Books, 2021.

Oshinsky, David M. *Polio: An American Story*. New York: Oxford University Press, 2005.

Skloot, Rebecca. *The Immortal Life of Henrietta Lacks*. New York: Crown, 2010.

Wadman, Meredith. *The Vaccine Race: Science, Politics, and the Human Costs of Defeating Disease*. New York: Viking, 2017.

CHILDREN'S BOOKS

While infants are unable to understand what's happening during vaccinations, young children, as well as adolescents, are often empowered by understanding why they need vaccines and what will happen at the vaccine visit. In addition, when parents are comfortable with and confident in their decisions related to their children's vaccines, the children tend also to be more comfortable and confident. For this reason, you may want to check out some books that describe vaccines:

- The University of Virginia created a collection of more than three hundred books addressing not only vaccines but also a variety of other topics that may be helpful for children, such as managing fear and anxiety, processing traumatic events, and grief and loss: https://guides.lib.virginia.edu/pandemicchildrensbooks.
- The Vaccine Education Center at Children's Hospital of Philadelphia offers "Vaccine Resources for Kids and Teens," which includes book recommendations and other resources: https://www.chop.edu/centers-programs/vaccine-education-center/resources/vaccine-resources-kids-and-teens.

WEBSITES AND MOBILE APPLICATIONS

For more information about vaccines and related topics, including opportunities to submit your own questions about vaccines, check out these resources:

- *Vaccines on the Go,* a free mobile app for iOS and Android devices: vaccine.chop.edu/mobileapp
- Centers for Disease Control and Prevention: https://www.cdc.gov/vaccines
  - ○ Vaccines for Children Program (VFC), program to get qualified children vaccinated for free: https://www.cdc.gov/vaccines/programs/vfc/parents/index.html
- Hilleman Film: https://hillemanfilm.com/

- National Foundation for Infectious Diseases: https://www.nfid.org/immunization
- Vaccinate Your Family: https://vaccinateyourfamily.org
- Vaccine Education Center at Children's Hospital of Philadelphia: https://vaccine.chop.edu
- Vaccine Information You Need (from Immunize.org): https://vaccineinformation.org
- Vaccine Makers Project: https://vaccinemakers.org/
- Voices for Vaccines: https://www.voicesforvaccines.org
- World Health Organization: https://www.who.int/health-topics/vaccines-and-immunization

ABOUT THE AUTHORS

PAUL A. OFFIT, MD

Paul A. Offit, MD, is the director of the Vaccine Education Center at Children's Hospital of Philadelphia, as well as the Maurice R. Hilleman Professor of Vaccinology and a professor of pediatrics at the Perelman School of Medicine at the University of Pennsylvania. He is the recipient of many awards, including the J. Edmund Bradley Prize for Excellence in Pediatrics from the University of Maryland Medical School, the Young Investigator Award in Vaccine Development from the Infectious Diseases Society of America, and a Research Career Development Award from the National Institutes of Health. Dr. Offit has published more than 170 papers in medical and scientific journals in the areas of rotavirus-specific immune responses and vaccine safety. He is also the co-inventor of the rotavirus vaccine, RotaTeq, recommended for universal use in infants by the Centers for Disease Control and Prevention in 2006 and by the World Health Organization in 2013. For this achievement Dr. Offit received the Luigi Mastroianni and William Osler Awards from the University of Pennsylvania School of Medicine and the Charles Mérieux

Award from the National Foundation for Infectious Diseases, and he was honored by Bill and Melinda Gates during the launch of their foundation's Living Proof Project for global health. In 2009, Dr. Offit received the President's Certificate for Outstanding Service from the American Academy of Pediatrics. In 2011, he received the David E. Rogers Award from the American Association of Medical Colleges and the Odyssey Award from the Center for Medicine in the Public Interest, and he was elected to the Institute of Medicine of the National Academy of Sciences. In 2012, Dr. Offit received the Distinguished Medical Achievement Award from the College of Physicians of Philadelphia. In 2013, he received the Maxwell Finland Award for Scientific Achievement from the National Foundation for Infectious Diseases and the Distinguished Alumnus Award from the University of Maryland School of Medicine. In 2015, Dr. Offit won the Lindback Award for Distinguished Teaching from the University of Pennsylvania and was elected to the American Academy of Arts and Sciences. In 2016, he won the Franklin Founder Award from the city of Philadelphia, the Porter Prize from the University of Pittsburgh School of Public Health, the Lifetime Achievement Award from the Philadelphia Business Journal, and the Jonathan E. Rhoads Medal for Distinguished Service to Medicine from the American Philosophical Society. In 2018, Dr. Offit received the Gold Medal from the Sabin Vaccine Institute, in 2019 the John P. McGovern Award from the American Medical Writers Association, and in 2020 the Public Educator Award from CHILD USA. In 2021, he was awarded the Edward Jenner Lifetime Achievement Award in Vaccinology from the Fifteenth Vaccine Congress and elected to the Baltimore Jewish Hall of Fame. In 2022, Dr. Offit received the Mentor of the Year Award from the Eastern Society for Pediatric Research and the Dean's Alumni Leadership Award from the University of Maryland School of Medicine. In 2023, he was elected to membership in the American Philosophical Society. Dr. Offit was a member of the Advisory Committee on Immunization Practices to the Centers for Disease Control and

Prevention, is currently a member of the Food and Drug Administration's Vaccine Advisory Committee, and is a founding advisory board member of the Autism Science Foundation and the Foundation for Vaccine Research. He is also the author of eleven medical narratives: *The Cutter Incident: How America's First Polio Vaccine Led to Today's Growing Vaccine Crisis* (2005); *Vaccinated: One Man's Quest to Defeat the World's Deadliest Diseases* (2007), for which he won an award from the American Medical Writers Association; *Autism's False Prophets: Bad Science, Risky Medicine, and the Search for a Cure* (2008); *Deadly Choices: How the Anti-vaccine Movement Threatens Us All* (2011), which was selected by Kirkus Reviews and Booklist as one of the best nonfiction books of the year; *Do You Believe in Magic? Vitamins, Supplements, and All Things Natural: A Look Behind the Curtain* (2013), which won the Robert P. Balles Prize in Critical Thinking from the Center for Skeptical Inquiry and was selected by National Public Radio as one of the best books of 2013; *Bad Faith: When Religious Belief Undermines Modern Medicine* (2015), which was selected by the *New York Times Book Review* as an "Editor's Choice" book in April 2015; *Pandora's Lab: Seven Stories of Science Gone Wrong* (2017), which was nominated for Best Science and Technology Book of 2017 by Goodreads; *Bad Advice: Or Why Celebrities, Politicians, and Activists Aren't Your Best Source of Health Information* (2018); *Overkill: When Modern Medicine Goes Too Far* (2020); *You Bet Your Life: From Blood Transfusions to Mass Vaccinations—The Long and Risky History of Medical Innovations* (2021), which was nominated for the Phi Beta Kappa Award in Science; and *Tell Me When It's Over: An Insider's Guide to Deciphering COVID Myths and Navigating Our Post-pandemic World* (2024).

CHARLOTTE A. MOSER, MS

Charlotte A. Moser, MS is the co-director of the Vaccine Education Center at Children's Hospital of Philadelphia. Ms. Moser holds a bachelor's degree in biology and a master's degree in science and health communication. She has published numerous scientific papers in the areas of disease prevention, immunology of the intestinal tract, and vaccine attitudes and beliefs. As a co-founder of the Vaccine Education Center, Ms. Moser has spent more than two decades designing content and resources to explain the science of vaccines to families with questions about how vaccines work and vaccine safety. She is the creator of Parents PACK, a program of the Vaccine Education Center that communicates with parents through a website, mobile app, and monthly email newsletter, and a co-creator of Vaccine Education Center programs for health care professionals and students of all ages. During the COVID-19 pandemic, Ms. Moser designed and implemented a dedicated web page, COVIDVaccineAnswers.org, to provide the public with access to the latest scientific information and a place to ask questions, and she oversaw the development of several video series about the COVID-19 vaccines. She also served on the COVID-19 Vaccine Advisory Committee of the Philadelphia Department of Public Health and the COVID-19 Vaccine Equity Committee at Children's Hospital of Philadelphia.

INDEX

inflammation, 38–39, 64–65, 189, 205–8, 219

influenza: cell-culture-based influenza vaccine, 192; death from, 189–90, 196–97; as disease, 187–88; to doctors, 29–30; FluMist vaccine, 11, 72; GBS and, 194–96, 280; hospitalization for, 30, 190–91, 197–98; HPV and, 19; immunity to, 6–7; inactivated influenza vaccine, 191; infections, 196–97; live, weakened influenza vaccine, 191–92, 194; meningococcus and, 5; pandemic, 177; pregnancy and, 119–20, 190; recombinant influenza vaccine, 192; research on, 198–200; rotavirus and, 91; RSV and, 198; symptoms of, 189–91; 3 to 6-year-old children and, 247–48; transmission of, 188, 196; in U.S., 197–98; vaccine, 40–41, 119–20, 191–97, 213, 250, 280, 306–12; vaccine schedules with, 306–12

information: on COVID-19, 208–11; on dengue, 277–78; about diphtheria, 141–43; about DTaP vaccine, 148–53; on hepatitis A, 239–40, 243–46; about hepatitis B, 138–40; on Hib, 177–78; on HPV, 271–72; on meningococcus, 251–52, 261–62; on mpox, 292–93, 297; for parents, 68; about pertussis,

145–48; on pneumococcus, 157–58; on polio, 184–86; on RSV, 303; science, 67–68; on shingles, 290–91; about tetanus, 143–45; VISs, 109

ingredients, in vaccines: adjuvants, 79–82; allergens, 70–75; animal products, 88–89; chemicals, 82–85; fetal cells, 85–88; preservatives, 75–79

inoculation sites, 110–11

insect cells, 12

insurance companies, 107

international travel, 107, 126–27

intestinal immunity, 25

intussusception, 37, 169

Investigational New Drug (IND) license, 16

IPV. *See* inactivated polio vaccine

Janssen/Johnson & Johnson vaccine, 86–87, 203, 206

Jenner, Edward, 3–4, 11, 292

Jeryl Lynn strain, 221

Jynneos, 294–97

Kinrix, 317

Langman, Rod, 101

lawsuits, 65, 67

licensure, for vaccines, 14, 16, 27–28, 98–99

lifestyle, 25–26, 34

live, weakened influenza vaccine, 191–92, 194

live, weakened measles vaccine, 221